Restoration of Breath

Consciousness Literature & the Arts 09

Restoration of Breath
Consciousness and Performance

SREENATH NAIR

Rodopi

Amsterdam - New York, NY 2007

Cover Design: Aart Jan Bergshoeff

The paper on which this book is printed meets the requirements of "ISO 9706:1994, Information and documentation - Paper for documents - Requirements for permanence".

ISBN: 978-90-420-2306-2
ISSN: 1573-2193

Printed in the Netherlands

To
Prof. K. Ayyappa Paniker

Contents

Acknowledgements

I would like to thank Dr. Daniel Meyer-Dinkgräfe, who supervised this research, and Guru Rajendra Siddha Yogi, who shared some valuable material and practical insights on Siddha Yoga meditation and *Restoration of Breath*, for their comments, observations and directions throughout in the development of this work, which inform several arguments in the thesis. I should thank Prof. Ralph Yarrow and Prof. David Ian Rabey for their thoughts and comments on the manuscript that helped me with some important modifications during this publication. Special thanks also must be recorded for the Department of Theatre, Film and Television studies for funding my studies at the University of Wales, Aberystwyth. I remember Prof. Ioan Williams, Head of the Department and Margaret Williams with gratitude for their interest and support to this research. I should also thank the members of staff in the Hugh Owen Library of the University of Wales Aberystwyth, the British Library in London and the admin staff in the Department of Theatre, Film and Television Studies at the University of Wales Aberystwyth. Many thanks also to Professor Michael Earley and Dr Diane Dubois of the School of Performing Arts, University of Lincoln, for arranging my teaching timetables such as to allow me the time to complete research for this thesis. I must give thanks to Arya Madhavan, my wife, for being so helpful, artistically and emotionally, during the entire process of the study: my observations on *Kudiyattam* in this book are largely informed by her.

Introduction

Breath is the flow of air between life and death. Breathing is an involuntary action that functions as the basis of all human activities, intellectual, artistic, emotional and physical. Breathing is the first autonomous individual action that brings life into being and the end of breathing is the definitive sign of disappearance. This book is an investigation of the dynamics of breath within the context of theatre. It explores the epistemological, psycho-physical and consciousness-related implications of breath for Western and Eastern acting and actor training, in four main chapters.

The first chapter explores theatre as a form of performativity and locates this type of performativity in the performer's body. On the basis of a definition of the terms and concepts of performativity and theatricality, I introduce the ways in which important thinkers of the 20th century, such as Heidegger, Foucault, Deleuze, Derrida and Irigaray made use of their respective understandings of the concept of performativity to develop their philosophies, especially the ways they suggest humans create meaning. In the course of the chapter I seek to demonstrate to what extent these thinkers consider performativity as an aspect of the body, and to what extent they consider breath as an important aspect of individual being.

Having established, in principle, the relevance of the body for performance, the relevance of breath for the body and thus the relevance of breath for performance in the first chapter, the second chapter proceeds to investigate traditional Western and Eastern knowledge and practice related to breath. Aristotle's *On Breath*, for instance, investigates the physiological and metaphysical functioning of breath in the body while examining pre-existent views of the ways in which breath has been conceived of and debated in the Greek natural philosophical tradition since Diogenes and Democritus. Aristotle elaborates these initial observations of the functioning of breath in the body further in his metaphysical speculations, arguing that the Soul and emotions are interconnected with the dynamics of breath. *Ch'i* is breath in the Chinese tradition. It is the air that we breathe in order to sustain vitality and energy in the body. According to the explanations provided by the *T'ai Ch'i* system, *Ch'i* operates the bipolar dynamics of *Yin* and *Yang*: what we breathe in is *Yin* and what we breathe out is *Yang*. *Ch'i* can exist without form and it can also exist in the form of a thought or action, the spiritual or material. The non-material states are pure energy, which is *Yang,* whereas the physical and material states are affiliated to *Yin*. According to the doctrines of Tao philosophy, establishing a natural cyclic equilibrium of these two forces is the strongest basis of good physical and mental health.

Breath is *prana* in Sanskrit. The theoretical and practical aspects of the term are discussed systematically and elaborately in various systems of knowledge in the Sanskrit tradition as a material phenomenon, which explains in depth our understanding of the conditions of linguistic meaning, visibility, appearance, human actions, voice and higher levels of consciousness. The integration of time and space is discussed extensively in *Sāmkhya* and *Yoga* in relation to breath, vitality and the cosmology of the body. According to *Sāmkhya,* the body's vital operations are performed by five forms of breaths called: *prana, apana, samana, udana and vyana*. These forms of breath are different modifications of the element of air, which incites the entire functioning of the system by bringing all the internal and external organs into action. *Yoga* proposes various techniques related to checking and changing of breathing in relation to allowing air flow predominantly through the left or right nostril for the purpose of changing the body's psycho-physical conditions. In several *Upanishads* we can see breath described in practical terms to experience higher states of consciousness. In the *Sangitaratnakara*, a text by Sarangadeva, the *Brahmarantra* is explained as the cerebral aperture, which is crucial to breath-related techniques in terms of exploring the dormant psychophysical energy levels of the body (I: II: 153c-155b). Agastiya's *Marmasastra* further explains and clarifies the bodily location, nature and functioning of the potential energy source of the body in more physiological terms. The South Indian Siva tradition and *Siddha Veda* offer a breath-related technique called *Restoration of Breath*, a system of twenty-four patterns of breathing by which the respiration can be completely internalised: the internalisation of breathing, in turn, alters individual consciousness.

The focus of Chapter three is the question of what, if any, of the aspects and dimensions of breath, explored in Chapter two, have been used in actor training both in the East and in the West, past and present. The chapter is divided into two major sections in which traditional Eastern and contemporary Western actor training will be discussed in terms of how breath has been integrated into practice. In the Eastern section I am mainly focusing on Keralan performance traditions, with particular emphasis on *Kudiyattam*, the Sanskrit theatre of India, mainly because I am familiar with this tradition and also have access to the material available locally. *Kudiyattam* is a highly stylised theatrical form with a strong emphasis on many years of systematic and complex training. Other areas of discussion in the same section will draw on the *Natyasastra*, the theatre manual describing the Indian concept of training and performance, with special emphasis on the concept of *rasa. Rasa* is best understood as the aesthetic delight experienced by the audience as the result of a theatrical event. In the section on contemporary Western actor training I shall focus mainly on the 20th century. Artaud does not create a practical training method, but in his writings we see accounts of some systems based on breath. I will refer to these as they become relevant in my discussions of the role breath plays in the theory and practice of Copeau, Stanislavski, Grotowski and Lecoq. I shall also look at some recent approaches like John Martin's intercultural training, Phillip Zarrilli's training method based on *Kalarippayattu* and Susanna Bloch's Alba Emoting.

The first three chapters of the book demonstrate the relevance of the breath for the body and of the body for performance (Chapter one), explore the ways breath has been understood across the history of ideas in West and East (Chapter two) and to what extent the available knowledge about breath has been used in the contexts of acting and actor training (Chapter three). Chapter four focuses in depth on a phenomenon that will have emerged, albeit implicitly, across the first three chapters: the body and breath cannot be understood without reference to consciousness. The relationship between embodied breath and consciousness is therefore at the centre of Chapter four. I provide information about contemporary consciousness studies and within that general context I compare a number of relevant specific models of consciousness that together serve the purpose of explaining the relationship between consciousness and breath. The book ends with a conclusion, in which I summarize my findings.

Chapter One
The Location of Breath

The intention of this chapter is to locate breath in the current discussions of performativity. Where is breath located and how does it function as the fundamental source of the production and reception of meaning and theatrical expression? Starting from these questions, this chapter explores the current discussions of theatricality and performativity, demonstrating how these concepts provide the context for interrelations between body, breath and meaning.

1.1 Theatricality and Performativity

The idea of theatricality has been identified with both the Greek idea of *mimesis* and the Latin concept of *theatrum mundi.*[1] Similarly, Sanskrit poetics in general and the *Rasa* theory in particular offer detailed descriptions of the concept and application of theatricality in performance as well as in literature and other arts. In the Greek classical tradition, according to Postlewait and Davis, the term *theatricality* has been used as *mimesis* "…to describe the gap between reality and its representation."[2] It has also been used to describe a different mode of perception by which the everyday reality is exceeded by its representation. It means that the mimetic representation transforms individual consciousness from the daily to extra-daily. For Plato, *mimesis* attempts to evoke the "factual" or real world but cannot capture it because "the real" is not located in "the visual and tangible conditions"[3] of the material world. Hence, theatre produces illusive *mimesis* that is "twice-removed" from the true or pure realm of the real. This "mimetic product" posits an empirical link between the perceiver and what is being represented, but this relation is always simply a "rhetoric feat" of similarity, never "sameness."[4] Thus, Plato disapproves of theatrical *mimesis* because the theatre may imitate life, but like a metaphor, the re-presentation is always removed from the real. Plato's argument has proved to be a strong foundation for the further development of antitheatrical attitudes in Western thought.

The concept of *lila* proposed by the Vedanta school of Indian philosophy implies a different idea of theatricality. According to Sankara, the notable proponent of the Vedanta school, the relation between the manifest world and the immaterial unmanifest *Brahman* operates through a 'playfulness' called *lila*. *Lila* refers to a process of the emergence of the physical world from the unmanifest that exists within the flow of time. Sankara explains *lila* in terms of the concept of *maya*. In the *Brahmasūtrabhāsya*, Sankara asserts that *maya* consists of two qualities: creative power and illusion.[5] Our perception of the world and the knowledge that we derive from this perception are the results of these two qualities: each perception is coloured by imagination and memory that together create the appearance of the world. Therefore, the appearance of the world is unreal (*avidya)*, in the sense that it is always in the process of transformation; our notion or impression, even our experience of the world's permanency, according to Sankara, is created by our false impressions and ignorance of the 'real' dynamics of microcosmic functioning. This process is called *lila*. "Creation" of any sort is essentially a "*lila*", a "free and a spontaneous *play*" by means of which the unmanifest (*Brahman)* is revealed and conceived through a process of infinite existence. *Lila* refers to theatricality, in a more subtle and complex manner, as playfulness and as the process of making and pursuing meaning out of a process in which forms emerge and submerge in the flow of time.

From current discussion of theatricality, we can derive, at least, two distinct uses of the term:

1. The fundamental characteristics of the production and reception of meaning of any event in the widest philosophical sense.

2. The essential performance qualities of any dramatic performance at any time or place, which is largely applicable to the communicative nature of art and literature.

Contemporary philosophers and theatre critics have employed the term in both ways to explain the functioning of the communicative nature embedded in human discourse.

Willmar Sauter argues that the term *theatrical* is widely used to describe a variety of situations and behaviours that often have nothing to do with theatre. For instance, graduation ceremonies, dancing, funerals and a politician's speech might be described as theatrical.[6] Sauter shows the use of the term in a performance situation saying that the concept of *theatricality* was developed as a modernist alternative to realism, and has been presented and debated in cultural, linguistic fields of study. As a critical concept, the term "…meant to represent the essential or possible characteristics of theatre as an art form and as a cultural phenomenon."[7] This approach offers critical tools to analyse the essential nature of making meaning within a performance, investigating how performance elements like movement, action, words, lines, objects, body and signs create emotional and cognitive experiences. As Roland Barthes noted, theatricality "…is theatre-minus-text, it is a density of signs and sensations built up on stage starting from the written argument."[8] Barthes locates theatricality in the fields of signs and codes of a performance. Scholars like Anne Ubersfeld criticised that Barthes is limiting the divergent communicative nature of performance when he insists on the idea that each stage performance has "three domains of referentialization: the dramatic text, itself (reflexive), and the natural world"[9] carrying emotive, connotative, referential, metalinguistic and poetic functions.

Erika Fisher-Lichte edited a range of articles in *Theatre Research International* aiming to clarify some classical and even more contemporary discussions on the concept of theatricality:

> Theatricality may be defined as a particular mode of using signs or as a particular kind of semiotic process in which particular signs (human beings and objects of their environment) are employed as signs of signs—by their producers, or their recipients. Thus a shift of the dominance within the semiotic function determines when theatricality appears. When the semiotic function of using signs as signs of signs in a behavioural, situational, or communication process is perceived and received as dominant, the behaviour, situational, or communication process may be regarded as theatrical. Moreover, since this shift of the dominant is not an objective given but depends on certain pragmatic

> conditions, "theatricality," in the end, appears to be no more than a floating signifier in an endless communication process. This is to say that the term theatricality necessarily remains defuse; as a concept, it becomes indistinct, if not void.[10]

Her emphasis is on a process of communication between presence and its perception. Here, theatricality is not only a pragmatic configuration of the conditions of cognition but relates to "floating signifiers" in the process of communication, which do not have any definite meaning until they are perceived by an onlooker. The meaning of theatricality, therefore, is closely associated with perception of the presence of things including the physical acts that shape an event. Thus, theatricality is a process of communication.

Conceptualising theatricality as a process of communication, Fisher-Lichte uses the term *performativity* in contrast to *theatricality* as a much larger concept. Critics like Carlson (1990; 1996), Kirby (1982; 1987) and Marranca (1977) insist that since the term theatricality, from a semiotic point of view, is understood as "a relation between sign and reference", it falls into the critical legacy of structuralist interpretations; whereas performativity as a concept "disrupts" and "denies" those relations that invite deconstructionist notions:[11] performativity as a concept, rather than asserting a specific hermeneutic meaning between sign and reference, indicates the ways in which a particular meaning is derived through its perception. Post-structuralist theories have emphasised the processes of reading and reception in order to locate the production of meaning rather than depending on any given interpretive meaning. The implications of these theories in a theatrical situation focus on audience reception in its communication as a major reflective element that produces meaning. From this perspective, theatricality and performativity are not opposing concepts. As Josette Féral suggests, performativity is one of the elements of theatricality.[12] Any spectacle, she argues, is an interplay of both performativity and theatricality. This interplay can be identified in every aspect of theatre, ranging from the paradox of acting— that puts the actor's body into a state of ambiguity between representation and the 'real', the 'profound duality of body in performance'— to the 'spectator's act of recognition'. Furthermore, this interplay is the play of ambivalences of everyday space versus representational space and reality versus fiction. Borrowing the idea of spatial overlap from Sauter, Féral insists that the nature of theatricality is an interplay between the work on stage and its reception by the audience. For both Sauter and Féral, the definition of theatricality encompasses all of the performing arts, including dance, opera, performance art and theatre. Therefore, both theatricality and performativity are not opposing terms but closely interconnected concepts.

In the following sections, I use the word performativity, rather than theatricality, in order to address the larger meaning of the concept. Performativity is a concept that intends to explain the nature and function of the production and the reception of meaning in a theoretical as well as in a theatrical situation. The following sections of this chapter will closely look at the specific categories of performativity, in order to investigate the implications of psycho-physical elements involved in the performative process. This analysis is important to this chapter because the link between breath and performativity can be established only on the basis of these psycho-physical categories.

1.2 Performance Categories of Performativity

The concepts and categories of performativity, particularly in a theatrical situation, have been discussed by a range of scholars from a variety of theoretical positions across the disciplines of social and cultural anthropology, linguistics, semiotics and phenomenology in order to formulate the notion of performativity as a critical term.

The concept of performativity is widely used in contemporary theoretical discourse, ranging, in various contexts, from philosophy via performance to linguistics and gender studies. Jacques Derrida and Judith Butler use the term as a complex process of citations through which identity is constructed *iteratively*, in the sense that meaning and identity are produced through a constant interplay between the reader and the act of reading. Foucault uses *performativity* as a field of discourse out of which the meaning of the individual self is formulated and controlled by various invisible power relations in history. Paul de Man's demonstration of deconstruction in reading is based on performativity as a textual strategy, "a radical estrangement between the meaning and the performance of any text."[13] In Austin, the relation between *speech* and *act* operates on the level of the interrelations between act and identity. Peggy Phelan refers to Austin's linguistic performativity as an important tool to understand the temporal dimension of performance, which only exists in the present.[14] As Phelan puts it:

> Performance cannot be saved, recorded, documented or otherwise participate in the circulation of representations of representation: once it does so, it becomes something other than performance.[15]

In this sense, performance occurs over a time that cannot be repeated. A performance can be repeated, but each repetition will be "different" from the previous one. For Phelan, this temporal realization of a theatrical situation's presentability is a performance's inherent performative quality. Thus performativity, as explained by Phelan, is a temporal act taking place in the 'here' and 'now' between the performer and the spectator, which cannot be reproduced or preserved. Richard Schechner, from a performance studies point of view argues that *performativity*, in a broader sense, is performance itself: the elements which constitute an event of performance such as any construction of social reality including gender and race, the restored behaviour quality of performances and the complex relationship of performance to its audience, all share common features with how the term is understood critically in other systems of knowledge.[16] The following is the brief review of those categories summarized and extended by Sauter based on the existing definitions of the term.[17]

1.2.1 Definition

Conferring a *metaphoric* meaning onto the notion of performativity, according to Erving Goffman, is one of the most popular ways of understanding the term: theatre is a metaphor of social behaviour. In this view, a theatrical performance as an event is metaphorically framed and hence, "how people enter the stage of life, how they approach the footlights to be exposed to the public, what they do behind the wings…" are the major concerns of this analysis. Anthropologist Victor Turner and philosopher Bruce Wilshire share similar views and have studied various other dimensions of the same concept in order to develop the idea of performativity as a critical term.[18] The limitation, according to Sauter, to this metaphorical approach is that most of these scholars have taken traditional domestic drama enacted in a naturalistic style on an American Broadway stage or in a BBC family series as the model for their analysis; in this sense, they have not either problematized nor investigated performativity in a broader and thus in its true sense. Rather, they reduced the notion of performativity to something that is pretended, which has to be analysed anthropologically between the two concepts of social drama and everyday life. Richard Schechner and Eugenio Barba are the major theoretical contributors of the anthropological approaches in Western academia and theatre scholarship. Despite Sauter's criticism, anthropological approaches of Schechner and Barba seem to have some significant contributions to contemporary performance research. Their approaches initially mobilise a terminological and methodological exploration in the area of academic studies of performance. Secondly, anthropological approaches to performance initiated a multicultural practice of research and performance in the contemporary theatrical scene.

The second definition of *performativity* is *descriptive*. It is mainly derived from the writings of Barthes, George Fuchs, Patrice Pavis and Hans-Thies Lehmann. Within this definition performativity is not what the text represents on the stage but rather it is the *mise-en-scène*, the result of the combination of the various other theatrical activities and signs, the theatrical configuration of the text that is mostly dealt with by the director. This approach borrowed theoretical assumptions from semiology and reception theory in order to clarify the symbolic nature of theatre communication. For instance, when Fischer-Lichte says that performativity is a "particular mode of using signs"[19] and therefore, theatrical signs are always signs of signs, she conforms to the descriptive notion of performativity from a semiotic point of view.

The third definition of performativity is binary; its key proposition is to establish strong aesthetic positions against naturalism in order to rescue the foundational characteristics of theatre related to the body, image and sounds that mark a significant departure from the most common traditional understanding of theatre as a verbal narrative. Starting from the works of the Russian Avant-garde in the early twentieth century, the conventional role assigned to theatre as a place where 'reality' is depicted is questioned by critics who have new ideas about and approaches to production. As a result, serious enquiries about the nature of performativity have been initiated and those enquiries have led to the radical proposition that rather than being loyal to 'reality', theatre should become a 'reality' of its own. This view has in turn brought about stylistic experiments in relation to production. Edward Gordon Craig and Antonin Artaud, according to Sauter, share the legacy of this idea of performativity.

The fourth category of performativity Sauter discusses is *epochal:* to convey the idea of performativity as a cultural concept. According to this view, performativity is a very difficult and complex phenomenon because each *epoch* develops different ideas on what theatre is, depending on the relevant cultural and historical situations. Sauter is sceptical about his fourth category: "if the concepts of theatricality change from epoch to epoch and from culture to culture, there might nevertheless be a common axis along which the definitions and concepts travel."[20] He argues that performativity can be regarded

1. as part of the performance on stage
2. as a specific style of theatrical presentation and
3. as a mode of perception.

He emphasises the "necessity of the physical presence of both the performer and the spectator as a prerequisite of theatricality."[21] In other words, no matter how we define the concepts or critical terms *theatricality* in the specific context of the theatre, or indeed *performativity* in the wider sense, they mainly consist of the interactive or self- reflexive processes of the production of meaning as a conscious "otherness" between the performance and its spectators. The awareness of having any kind of meaning is always related to the physical presence of bodies and other animate and inanimate objects in time and space. Thus the idea is that each physical presence is marked by our subjective reflections of various kinds and therefore, human cognitive and emotional processes are mediated by these two phenomenal factors: physical presence of the object and subjective reflections of it. In this sense, performativity as an interactive process between presence and perception constitutes the basic configuration of consciousness and meaning.

1.2.2 Enacted Performativity

Physical enactment is another key aspect to performativity. Sauter classifies theatrical actions that form the basis of performativity as follows[22]:

1. *Exhibitory actions*: physical presence showing the individual presence without doing any particular actions. These actions also include subsequent mental conditions but those are not expressed.

2. *Encoded actions*: the actions that suggest expressive meanings. They encompass gestures and postures mediated by movements that are underpinned by individual, cultural and aesthetic conditions. Movements are partly conditioned by 'natural' behaviours and partly by cultural patterns; it is difficult to distinguish involuntary movements from consciously expressive gestures. Encoded actions are intended to signify something which is beyond the directly perceived appearance of those actions.

3. *Embodied actions*: Exhibitory and encoded actions do not necessarily suggest a symbolic level, which is inherited in embodied actions. Embodied actions are actions in which the performer chooses to convey consciously something beyond what he/she does. From a performance point of view, embodied actions are pretended ones –the fictive dimension of a performance.

Sauter's primary concern in this classification of the physical enactment is to reemphasise the role of the body in the production of meaning.

1.2.3 Reception and Performativity

Audience reception is considered as a key theatrical category of performativity and Sauter offers a classification of four categories of audience reception in the context of theatre performance:

1) reflections of prior experiences
2) emotional reactions
3) cognitive reactions and
4) value judgements.[23]

Cognitive processes take place and intermingle with emotions in a theatrical situation. Information transmitted from a performance is received and processed intellectually, on the one hand and on the other hand, each moment of cognition stimulates subsequent emotions. The interaction between these two modes of reactions—the intuitive and emotional, and the cognitive—in the spectator's mind are vital elements that produce a theatrical event.

From a spectator's point of view, prior experiences produce expectations, preferences and prejudices in the process of perception of a theatrical event. They have a strong impact on both the cognitive and the emotional reactions during and after the performance. Value judgement is another important factor that co-exists with prior experiences and finally shapes the feeling and opinion of the actuality of a theatrical experience. In fact, prior experience and value judgement are the elements of perceptual reactions that figurate audience's direct responses to the performance through the multiple channels of reception.

Cognition and emotions are the major components of an audience's response to a performance. In a performance, the spectator's emotional process starts with a stimulus from the stage that they, consciously or unconsciously, analyse, compare to their own experiences and the perceived experiences of others, evaluate and finally transform into an adequate feeling or a cognitive action through aesthetic responses.[24] In addition to this, the perception of a stage performance causes:

1. automatic responses that are gradually processed into cognitive knowledge.
2. persistent feelings, which remain active during an entire performance.[25]

Theatrical experience, then, is the interplay between emotional and intellectual responses while confronting a set of encoded theatrical actions on stage. It is transferred through physical actions and received by the spectators against the background of their life experiences. The spectator realises the fact that the actions presented on stage are pretended ones because those actions are the actions of the others, the actors and the fictive characters. The performance also makes the spectator aware of the fact that the actions are of a different kind, suggesting something symbolically, which are open to interpretation on both emotional and intellectual levels. The bodies in performance are biological bodies placed in praxis. At the same time those bodies are the bodies of the 'others'. Performance is a physical 'reality', which can be defined empirically. At the same time, there is an inherent subjective element in this process of reception that transforms all the materiality related to a performance into fictional terms.

According to Sauter's classification, there are three modes of audience re-actions parallel to his own three classifications of theatrical actions, which are: *sensory*, related to exhibitory actions; *artistic,* related to encoded actions; and *symbolic*, related to embodied actions.[26] The *sensory* level of reception indicates the initial perception of a stage personality whereas the *artistic* level relates more to the aesthetic dimensions of a theatre presentation. The *symbolic* is the fictional level, which, according to Sauter, goes beyond the level of any methodological understandings of cultural empiricism. On a *symbolic* level, theatre communication indicates various other possibilities of subjective interaction of spectators with the physical elements of performance through extra-theatrical and intra-theatrical scales,": the understanding of expressive means either comes from outside the performance… [from a prior subjective experience] or comes from within the theatre and its own conventions."[27] Theatrical experience is not limited either to physical appearance or to subjective reflections, but it comprises both.

Performativity, as a concept, refers to this 'play of ambivalence' between the objective world and its subsequent subjective reflections. Performativity is the inherent nature of a process that operates in between the objective world of theatricality and its reflexive act of perception in order to create meaning and consciousness. Both the material world of theatricality and its reflexive meaning as perception are largely influenced and defined by cultural and historical factors.

Our understanding of space, time and the objective world is related to the perceptual faculties of our body and its inherent libidinal energy that mobilises movement and intentional actions. This movement eventually leads to pleasure and other experiences of various kinds. Therefore, the cognitive and emotional experiences in and of a performance are mediated by perception: performance of any kind consists of its double: praxis and perception, the physical aspect of the performance including enactment and the spectators' subjective reception. Hence, the theatrical experience can be said to be an act of perception in praxis. Ittelson offers a clear distinction of this functional aspect of the act of perception with reference to two other phenomenological approaches.[28] The *stimulus-response* approach attempts to define perception in terms of *observable characteristics* of the stimulus and the response. These two approaches grow out of two different philosophical ways of thinking. The first mode is that of the 'idealists' who concentrate on the thoughts and feelings of their own experience, while the second represents the 'realists' who are concerned only with the observable objects and events of the external world. Eventually, the first view culminates in that of the solipsist, who believes that there is nothing outside of his/her own inner experience, the latter view in that of the behaviourist who believes that there is nothing inside of his. As Ittelson puts it:

> The functional definition tries to bridge the gap between these divergent views by specifying the perceptual process in terms of the relationship of that particular process to the total life functioning of the individual. A functional approach is by its very nature future oriented and goal-directed.[29]

According to Ittelson's classification, the functional definition puts the actor as well as the spectator into a 'real' life-like situation and considers him as he actually appears in concrete living. Therefore, it is clear that the individual acts in any situation in terms of the ways he perceives the situation. Perception, then, becomes a crucial process intimately involved in the effective psycho-physical functioning of the individual in the spatio-temporality of the objective world. This functional approach towards the phenomenology of perception is useful to understand the ways in which performativity operates in a theatrical situation through multiple channels of transmission.

Indian aesthetic theory offers a different understanding of the performative importance of audience reception. The key concept in the Indian aesthetic theory presented in the *Natyasastra* is *rasa*, which is understood as the performer's as well as the spectator's aesthetic experience. The concept is phrased in the *Natyasastra* in the form of a *sutra*, a short statement that is *vibhava-anubhava-vyabhicharibhava-samyogat rasa-nishpattih* (NS, 109). Meyer-Dinkgräfe provides the following rendering, based on Ghosh's translation: "Rasa is produced (*rasa-nishpattih)* from a combination (*samyogat)* of determinants (*vibhava*), consequence (*anubhava*), and transitory mental states (*vyabhicharibhava*)."[30] According to the critical legacy of Sanskrit poetics, *vibhava* is again classified into two: the *alambana vibhava* and the *udhipana vibhava*, the character-performer and the situation or the given circumstances. For example, in the context of erotic sentiment (*Sringara rasa)*, the lovers are the *alambana vibhava,* which literally means the base or reasons for determinants, the observable aspects of perception; and the fragrance of flowers and garlands, ornaments, senses of objects, going to a garden and enjoying there, seeing and hearing the beloved and playing with her/him are the *udhipana vibhava*, which literally means the stimulants of determinants, the stimulus aspects of perception. Consequents (*anubhava*) are defined as means of histrionic representation.

In the above example, clever movements of eyes, glances, soft and delicate movements of the limbs and sweet words and the like are the functional aspects of perception. *Vyabhicahri bhavas* are explained as thirty-three transitory mental states like intoxication, anxiety, envy, depression, dreaming etc… that are the experience of *rasa* as the result of these levels of perception. This phenomenological approach of the *rasa* theory to the nature of theatrical experience is firmly based on the following assumptions:

1. Acts of perception always present themselves through concrete individuals dealing with concrete situations. They also can be studied in terms of *transactions* in which they can be observed.

2. Perceiving is done by a particular person from his own position in space and time and his own combination of experiences and needs. It is a field of *personal behaviours.*

3. Since the act of perception is interposed by the personal behaviours, each act of perception attributes certain aspects of personal experience to an environment, which we may believe exists independent of experience. It is a characteristic perception of *externalisation.*

To summarise both the findings of this section, we can say that the interaction between the performer's actions and the spectator's reactions is characterized by three interactive levels of theatrical communication: sensory, artistic and symbolic. These levels can only be activated through the process of performance and only this process facilitates performativity. According to Sauter, performativity is something that takes place *between* actions and reactions. He disagrees with Fischer-Lichte on her key argument that 'the use of signs' designates theatricality. Nor does he think that theatricality is a specific 'mode of perception' as Burns uses the term. Rather he focuses on both perspectives as "…both actions which become signs and reactions through which these signs are perceived in a special way."[31] Therefore, the question of performativity as a communicative process, for Sauter, is a process of various actions taking place *between* the performer's *exhibitory, encoded* and *embodied* actions and the emotional and intellectual reactions of the spectator. For Sauter performativity consists in psycho-physical movements taking place in *between* the presented actions and their perception in a performance situation. Sauter's emphasises the psycho-physical bases of the role of performativity as an interactive process between representation (performance) and its perception (audience reception). The embodied actions as well as the act of perception are activities related to the actor's and the spectator's physical bodies. The following conclusions can be derived from this section:

1. Theatricality and performativity are terms that refer to the communicative process within textual and performance situations.

2. Meanings, emotional as well intellectual, are produced through a performative interaction *between* signs and their reception.

3. Performativity is psycho-physical because the body as the embodiment of psycho-physical elements is the base for all our cognitive and emotional experiences.

If performativity includes embodied psycho-physicality in terms of the production and reception of meaning, what is the role of breath within it? I shall argue that theoretical explanations of performativity have more or less ignored the role of breath in understanding performativity. In the course of the thesis I aim to show the relevance of breath for performance, thus closing the currently existing gap. The following section in the chapter will first of all establish the epistemological link between breath and performativity.

1.3 Critical Categories of Performativity

The emphasis of performativity is a relatively recent phase of philosophical thinking in contemporary critical theory and scholarship, initiated by the post-war French thinkers through structural linguistics, phenomenology and psychoanalysis. This theoretical advancement constituted a rereading of the philosophical and aesthetic status of the classical notions of *mimesis* initially delineated by Plato and Aristotle, a concept developed further throughout in the history of philosophy. In the context of the role of performativity, I will look at the most recent phase of critical thinking considering the works from Michel Foucault, Gilles Deleuze and Jacques Derrida. Artaud is equally important in this context, though he is not qualified as a philosopher as the other three. However, Artaud remains as the source of a radical thinking that is relevant not only to theatre practice but also to contemporary philosophy and this is the reason why Derrida paid homage to Artaud's life and works. Artaud is significantly important to this chapter because we can see Artaud establishing epistemological links between breath and performativity, in his monumental book, *Theatre and its Double.* The following sections demonstrate how performativity has been discussed in recent critical thinking.

1.3.1 Foucault and Event

In a short discussion of Deleuze's *Difference and Repetition*, Foucault examines three major methodologies of the recent past that attempt to conceptualize or define the nature of event: neopositivism, phenomenology, and the philosophy of history.[32] According to Foucault, neopositivism failed to grasp the distinctive level of the event because of its logical error that confuses the perception of an event with a state of things: for neopositivism, an event is a material process attached explicitly to physicalism. Phenomenology reconsidered the idea of event in terms of meaning. For phenomenology, the world is a primary signification structured around the self indicating in advance where the event might occur. Foucault argues that phenomenology is "the grammar of the first person" and "the metaphysics of consciousness"[33] in which the meaning never coincides with an event. The event does not exist in phenomenology: rather it appears as the signifiers of meaning and therefore, what exists in phenomenology is only the self as a reflection of the world: world exists through the self. Finally, in the philosophy of history, the event is "enclosed" in a "cyclical pattern of time"[34]: it treats the present as framed by the past and future: "the present is a former future where its form was prepared and the past, which will occur in the future."[35] This pattern of time always preserves "the identity of its content,"[36] which means that the present exists in a "logic of essence"[37] that links present to past through memory and to future through concepts as a knowledge regained for the future. Thus, the philosophy of history proposes a cyclical concept of time and therefore Foucault suggests that this time is static and unable to grasp an event.

Foucault considered event not as a concept but strictly as a temporal force existing in the present time, which cannot be controlled or determined by any methods of programmes. An event cannot be defined when it occurs in the present time. The event can only be narrated after its occurrence, which certainly determines the specificity and uniqueness as well as the linguistic *iterability* of the event. As Paul Patton suggests, "events are incorporeal transformations which are expressed in language but attributed to bodies and state of affairs... It does not simply represent the world but intervenes in it."[38] An event, therefore, is an active process that takes place in the structural dimension of space and temporality. As Foucault conceived it, event as an irreducible temporal force disorients the notion of "pure" present. By reading Deleuze, Foucault formulates his thoughts successfully, which help us to understand the nature of event. Commenting on Deleuze's intellectual contribution to the history of Western thought, Foucault argues that what Deleuze offers to resolve this methodological error is not a phenomenology of signification based on the subject, but rather a thought of "the present infinitive."[39] The latter is not the rising up of the conceptual future in a past essence, but, a moment of being continuously in the present time. As Deleuze explains it:

> Just as the present measures the temporal realization of the event—the event in turn...has no present. It rather retreats and advances in two directions at once, being the perpetual object of a double question: what is going to happen? What has just happened? The agonizing aspect of the pure event is that it is always and at the same time something which has just happened and something about to happen...the living present happens and brings about the event. But the event nonetheless retains an eternal truth...The event is that no one ever dies, but has always just died or is always going to die...Each event is the smallest time...because it is divided into proximate past and immediate future...But it is also the longest time...because it is endlessly subdivided.[40]

Deleuze's analysis of an event as an endless seriality of occurrences brought new dimensions of thought into the post-phenomenological strands in Western philosophy. This temporal dimension of an event as "present infinitive" is the potential ground for performativity. What both Foucault and Deleuze speak about is the irreducible temporality of performativity. Event is the smallest unit of time, which is taking place in time. This, in fact, is the act or the performance, or an occurrence on which the whole concept of performativity is built. It is also the smallest unit of knowledge or sense of being. In other words, cognition or the sense of being is the results of the process of this occurrence in time; that is performativity. Let us look at this aspect in detail as to how Deleuze formulates this idea of performativity in connection with theatre as a major core of this intellectual activity.

1.3.2 Deleuze and Repetition

Deleuze's concept of repetition is the modernist revision of *mimesis*. With the thinkers of modernity, *mimesis* turns into repetition as a temporal dimension of representation and reality. Martin Heidegger, for instance, when discussing Platonic *mimesis*, insists that the idea is directed towards *truth* but based on the *distance* from it. This means that *mimesis* is based on the idea that artists cannot reproduce truth as similarity. According to Heidegger, to associate *mimesis* with "primitive" imitation is a wrong reading, rather, for him, it is a question of "doing after: production that comes afterwards. The *mimesis* is in its essence situated and defined through distance."[41] Following Heidegger, Hans Georg Gadamer also suggests *mimesis* as a "productive relation to knowledge and truth"; as he argues that "recognition" is the closest word that characterizes "a mimetical sense of knowledge."[42] Both Heidegger and Gadamer suggest that *mimesis* is productive rather than imitative. This definition of *mimesis* refers to a temporal dimension, which is closer to the concept of repetition that many of the modern thinkers like Nietzsche and Freud used. Therefore, the modern notion of *mimesis* is always "the meeting-place of two opposing but connected ways of thinking, acting and making: similarity and difference."[43]

According to Deleuze, Kierkegaard and Nietzsche introduce the concept of movement in philosophy. They are the ones who put metaphysics into motion, into action, which means that they redefined *cogito* in terms of time, a new representation of movement. *Cogito ergo sum,* or *I think, therefore I am,* is a canonical formulation about individual self consciousness by which Descartes explains the basic nature of the process of knowing. As he explained, the *cogito* proposes that I exist *in so far as* I am a thinking thing, *whatever that turns out to be*. Descartes thus establishes the supremacy of the ontological nature of the thinking subject.[44] In Descartes, the existence of the body is subjected to doubts due to the existence of thoughts. Cognition, therefore, is a binary split between the body and mind. Descartes, in this sense, rejects the fundamental interlocking dynamics between the body and mind operating on the temporal level of human existence. In its classical definition, representation is explained as mediation between perception and meaning, but for Kierkegaard and Nietzsche, representation works only in temporality, in movement, which are capable of affecting the mind outside of all representation. This very idea of representation as movement is close to theatre because performance as a world of signification is based on animation. As Deleuze suggests:

> Something completely new begins with Kierkegaard and Nietzsche. They no longer reflect on the theatre in the Hegelian manner. Neither do they set up a philosophical theatre. They invent an incredible equivalent of theatre within philosophy, thereby founding simultaneously this theatre of the future and a new philosophy.[45]

Both Kierkegaard and Nietzsche share the same philosophical views of movement in *cogito*, and it is because of the same reason they object to Hegel's allegedly false notion of movement, arguing that Hegel does not go beyond the notion of false movement, the "abstract logical movement of mediation."[46] Deleuze argues that Hegel remains in the world of "the reflected element of representation" between "the singular and the universal" only on the ground of an idea.[47] In order to clarify the historicity of the concept, Deleuze argues that Marx's criticism of Hegel originated from the same philosophical point of view. In other words, while considering history as a constant process, Marx incorporates this dynamics of movement at the centre of his thoughts. He believes that the events that change the world are always based on certain movements of dialectic inherent within the formation of history and hence there will be always a possibility of changes in the material conditions organized by specific historical moments. No human condition is static but constantly in motion, because in any historical situation the productive forces are always in action or in motion with each other. For Deleuze, this Marxian view of history is nothing but a theatrical idea and therefore, closer to repetition except for Marx's focus on binary opposition. In the sense, Marx believes that history is made from the dialectics of conflicts between working force and the capital force. Deleuze does not believe that the productive forces are always in opposition in history because there are other ways in which power operates through various performative practices, which include the linguistic, the cultural and the epistemological.

Deleuze argues that *repetition* as a movement is not an abstract idea but the movement that is essentially supported by the physical and psychic movements involved in the process of the production and reception of meaning. Repetition is not the representation of an ideal reality but the movement of *physis* and *psyche* exists constantly in time in the form of an occurrence. Deleuze further explains the links between theatre and repetition, establishing the physical and psychic kinesis working throughout in a performance. In his argument he refers to "the signs and masks through which the actor plays a role which plays other roles."[48] Deleuze is referring to the multiple possibilities of reception of a performance in which repetition, as a movement, brings the 'play' of theatrical signs: bodies, signs and various patterns of forms and colours repeat in a performance. Here, Deleuze emphasises the point that the production of meaning in a performance situation, fundamentally, derives from the kinesis of performance, not from any concept. He rejects the idea of the theatre as representation:

> The theatre of repetition is opposed to the theatre of representation, just as movement is opposed to the concept and to representation which refers it back to the concept.[49]

Representation is conceptual and repetition is psycho-physical, embedded in movement in time and space. As he further explains:

> In the theatre of repetition, we experience pure forces, dynamic lines in space which act without intermediary upon the spirit, and think it directly with nature and history, with a language which speaks before words, with gestures which develop before organized bodies, with masks before faces, with spectres and phantoms before characters—the whole apparatus of repetition as a 'terrible power'.[50]

While analysing the temporal dimension of meaning and consciousness within various philosophical systems of thought, Deleuze identified two recurring infinite elements that operate in the process of making sense of the world: 1) remembering and recognition and 2) memory and self-consciousness. According to Deleuze, memory is a temporal activity travelling back and forth between the appearance of an object and the re-cognition of its meaning. The links between a concept and its object are established by the dynamics of this double aspect, memory and self-consciousness. This relation is what is called 'representation' in a philosophical context. The very act of the movement of relating a concept to its object consists of similarity and difference at the same time, because in each repetition the object is perceived differently. In another sense, the comprehension of a concept always relates to the similarity of its object but at the same time the object is perceived differently. This means, each moment of understanding is the movement of repetition of *physis* and *psyche* in the world of difference infinitely repeated in time. As Deleuze explains the phenomenon, "repetition, thus appears as difference without a concept, repetition which escapes indefinitely continued conceptual difference."[51] It is the power of physical and psychic movement, the pure force repeating in time and space. According to Deleuze, theatre takes place fundamentally through repetition. To sum up, Deleuze's *repetition* is the psycho-physical movement that occurs in time and space as lived experience.

1.3.3 Derrida and Différance

Derrida's *différance* refers to a kind of temporal concept similar to *repetition* in relation to representation and meaning. As he explains the term in *Margins of Philosophy,* it is "neither a word not a concept" rather, it is temporization of consciousness.[52] As we have seen in the section *Foucault and Event*, the phenomenological understanding of consciousness/meaning is closely associated with the "presentation of the being-present," which means that the object is revealed through the presence of the self; without the presence of this self the world hardly exists outside of individual consciousness. Derrida believes that this notion of self as the centre of meaning, however, is the methodological error found in Husserl's phenomenology. This is the reason why Derrida's thought is known as the declaration of the end of phenomenology and hence, his methodology is known as the decentralization of thoughts as deconstruction. While engaged in this phenomenological deconstruction, Derrida has formulated his own phenomenological base by finding Heidegger at his starting point. The importance of the idea of time in Heidegger's philosophical writings is what attracts Derrida. In Heidegger's philosophical project, we could see time as an "interpretation of *time* as horizon for an understanding of Being,"[53] which means that the question of Being can be answered only in terms of time; and this *time* is *movement* according to Heidegger in his phenomenological "destruction" of the philosophical history of ontology. Therefore, Being in Heidegger, as Melberg quotes from his original German edition of *Sein und Zeit*, is the enigmatic movement of time, and this is the movement that makes *being* present in time. Being is always as present as it is concealed, always appearing and always in the act of withdrawing. Heidegger defines Being as presence as "what is being grasped in its Being as presence, for instance, is understood in relation to a definite mode of time, the present. The present time and the presence of time."[54] Being, for Heidegger, is a *play* of presence and absence in time "with its permanent movement" and the forward direction—into "nothingness"—of the movement. He also explains this inevitable movement forward to "nothingness" by using another term *Wiederholung*, which literally means *repetition*. Heidegger uses two more terms while explaining the nature of Being as an enigmatic movement forward: *Entschlossenheit* (resoluteness) and *Augenblick* (instant). As Melberg translates Heidegger's words, in "resoluteness (*Entschlossenheit*) the present is not only brought back from diversion in what is close and cared for, but will be held in the future and in having been."[55] The idea derived from this explanation of the movement of time, as Melberg paraphrases it, is the floating or the sequential time which is concentrated into an "instant" that reformulates or repeats the possibilities of the past and transports them into future. We see now that Heidegger's *Wiederholung* and Deleuze's *repetition* are similar concepts establishing the idea that individual consciousness in terms of reception and meaning is a temporal phenomenon embedded in physical as well as psychic movement.

Derrida's *différance* could be viewed as the development of Heideggerian Being but at the same time differs on various levels. As Derrida suggests, *différance* is both spatial difference and temporal displacement, which means that the meaning of the sign is revealed only within the "repetitive structure" of language and the "presence-of-the-present" is derived from repetition, and not the reverse. This is again the temporization of meaning that Derrida calls *iterability*.

Iterability derives, according to Derrida's etymological speculation, not only from the Latin *iter* (again) but also from *itara*, the *other* in Sanskrit.[56] It denotes "alterability in the singularity of the event," which means that a sign, in its being, always draws attention to its double meaning that includes difference: the thing is neither what it had been in the past nor what it would be in the future; rather it is what it is. The activity of the spatial and temporal displacement of a sign contains or conceals what is not present in it, which means, the displacement conceals the past within the presence in the form of absence: it is not the same. In this sense, each presence contains its "other": the invisible existence in the past. This is what Derrida calls *trace* and language as a sign is a trace on which the 'real' is absent. Therefore, reading, for Derrida, is an infinite repetition of signs within the structure of repetition that never fixes meaning but extends it in time by incorporating another occurrence of sign in space and in time. Hence, according to Derrida, consciousness and meaning are not a thing but an endless repetition of identification and difference in space and time in which each moment in an event carries the *previous* moment as *trace* inscribed in the presence as absence. This is the "dialectic of repetition", the endless process of deconstructing the "presence" and for Derrida, this act is the act of "tracing of *différances*" and "the concept of *play* keeps itself beyond its opposition, announcing, on the eve of philosophy and beyond it, the unity of chance and necessity in calculations without end."[57] Derrida admits the fact that the concepts of temporization and displacement are already explained by Nietzsche and Freud as "active" movements in metaphysics as well as in psychoanalysis as the function of thought and unconscious.[58] This brief demonstration of Derrida's philosophical ideas suggests that what he has explained through his various philosophical terms is referring to the performativity of meaning in a linguistic context. Derrida also brought performance into philosophy by defining temporal occurrences and the reader/onlooker as the perceptive self in order to deconstruct any fixed notions of meaning. This is the very nature of theatricality as meaning only emerges and submerges in the mind of the spectators through a constant play of signifiers including the body and its movements submitted to perception.

Derrida also made some reflections on theatre practice when he commemorated Artaud and it is highly essential to look at Artaud's idea of performativity in order to trace the epistemological ground between breath and performativity. Both Artaud and Derrida are interested in philosophy and theatre in their own ways. While Artaud attempts to explore the metaphysics in theatre, Derrida's intention was to perform philosophy through his *play* of the act of deconstruction. In the following section, I analyse briefly both approaches, the theatricality of philosophy and the philosophy of theatricality in order trace the whole argument offered in this chapter for further discussion.

1.3.4 Artaud and Breath

Artaud rejects representation in theatre in order to investigate the 'real' nature of the art. While doing this, he was, in fact, challenging the fundamental assumptions of *mimesis*, the imitative concepts of aesthetics developed in Western metaphysics since Plato and Aristotle. Artaud asks provocative questions related to body, gestures, movement, voice and breath, the entire physicality of body that has the potential of creating a theatrical meaning of its own, to re-establish a different poetry of "flesh" and "blood" which he called *cruelty*. To a large extent, Artaud's language, particularly the way he uses it to clarify his ideas and thoughts, is metaphorical and this is the major difficulty in understanding his theses. I do not want argue either that Artaud eventually ends up with the conflict between "madness" and "reason" without making much sense in what he has been discussing; or celebrating the idea of Derridian "closure" repeatedly in terms of representation, writing and meaning. Instead, my intention in this section is to investigate: 1) the conceptual ground of Artaud's rejection of representation 2) the nature of performativity that Artaud proposed and finally, 3) the role of breath in his theatre aesthetics.

Artaud points out that cruelty must not be taken in its literary sense of "merciless bloodshed, pointless and gratuitous pursuit of physical pain."[59] Rather, it is "the aspect of our own existence," whose existence is not defined by a particular historical time; rather, *time* in a current philosophical sense. Thus, Artaud is very clear in using this term as an image that is entwined with the very condition of being, which has always "been there": *cruelty* is neither an invention nor an "adjunct" of his thoughts. For Artaud, cruelty is a "hungering after life" and the "restless necessity" in the Gnostic sense of vortex, the "inescapability" of Being without which life could not continue. Artaud's views suggest the enigma of the presence of time as an never-ending movement in which the Self is revealed through *acts* by being at the edge of its motion. Artaud clarifies the link between consciousness, time and human act further, indicating that life is a constant process through which the meaning of Being is produced.

> There is no cruelty without consciousness, without the application of consciousness, for the latter gives practicing any act in life a blood red tinge, its cruel over tones, since it is understood that being alive always means the death of someone else.[60]

This enigma of being-in-present in time is characteristic of philosophical concepts developed by Nietzsche, Heidegger, Deleuze and Derrida, as discussed in earlier sections of this chapter. Artaud distinctively separates cruelty as consciousness and the application of it as *acts,* through which the sense of Being is established. Hence, cruelty, for Artaud, is the temporisation of meaning/consciousness and theatre; it is the living example of this philosophical view. Theatre for Artaud is based on *the magic act* which obeys this inescapability of being-in-present that permits "constant creation" in time and space. Artaud called this the *desire* that makes theatre possible, the desire for always being-in-present. This *desire* is the psycho-physical urge to be in the present, to be in consciousness: the underlying energy to all the emotional and cognitive processes. The failure of theatre, according to Artaud, is forgetting this *desire*, this temporal dimension that creates movement, gestures, sounds and other physical appearances relating to the body. This temporal and physical force is, in fact, beyond the structure of language and also the most important element that *plays* as "the transcendent aspect of the plot": without this physical force in time as presence, the plot will not transcend into experience. This temporal perspective provides a firm philosophical ground for Artaud to reject representation in theatre. It is very clear in this brief analysis why Artaud surpasses representation and reinforces the body in his theatre; it is simply because he rediscovered the ancient strength of *Oriental* theatre as the non-representational enactment of the physicality of the body constantly destined to be at the edge of time. Therefore, theatre is a continuous process and a vibrant movement in space and time that cannot be preserved or regained; for that reason. Artaud called it the *magical act*. It is *magical* because it is movement which cannot be captured in frozen time. It is also the fact that each moment in time is endlessly transformational: the present transforms into another present, not into future.

Artaud called this structure of time the "cosmic strictness" and the "relentless necessity." Both Artaud's philosophical ground and his views on the nature of theatricality could be understood by these temporal sequences, which is a common trend with many philosophers and critics of theatricality in recent history that we have been looking at in this chapter. Artaud's theatricality is not the frozen time of representation but an active time of repetition of the body in the present time. Repetition here is used not in its literal sense but in its philosophical sense, as either an event or a movement that is not repeatable in the same way twice. Derrida might argue in this context that each moment in the past is inscribed in the present as *trace* and that therefore there is no closure of space in which the traces could be re-presented, which means that one has no space outside representation and therefore it continues. Derrida argues that representation is time itself in the form of repetition and each presence in time refers to its existence in the past, the history of the presence that belongs to some another point of time in the past, from which there is no way of escaping. This Derridian rereading of Artaud remains as one of the most important intellectual debates of our time on and around the issues of representation, reality and consciousness. The question Derrida asks still remains unresolved by both Artaud and Derrida, as their unfinished projects, and my task here is to look at Artaud's views on representation in the light of Derrida's rejoinder to make sure that Artaud has not been misread by Derrida.

Derrida, in his careful reading of Artaud, agrees that "the theatre of cruelty is not a *representation*": it is "life" itself to the extent to which it is "unrepresentable". According to Artaud's words, "art is not the imitation of life, but life is the imitation of a transcendental principle which art puts us into communication with once again."[61] Derrida further clarifies Artaud's intention of resisting representation in the name of the body, arguing that the stage certainly "will no longer represent", since it will not operate as the "sensory illustration of a text already written." Artaud believes that the "stage will no longer operate as the repetition of the *present*" in the sense of re-presenting an already existing event. Derrida identifies two key concepts shaping Artaud's entire arguments: 1) repetition and 2) pure presence. In order to analyse Artaud's notions of repetition and pure presence, first of all Derrida clarifies Artaud's view on representation by saying that representation for Artaud is not the "surface of spectacle displayed for spectators". Rather what Artaud meant is the "representation that signifies an experience which produces its own space"[62].Artaud's representation is not re-presentation of a text or of an event that existed beforehand. It is the *presence* of visual objects that produce their own experience without any addition of an event or a text that pre-exists. Derrida argues that Artaud declared a "closure of representation" by prophesying an "original representation" which is a "pure presence" of experience. This Artaudian visible representation is directed against the "speech which eludes sight." Derrida is very clear about Artaud's intentions when he says Artaud will not perform any written text. This means that each speech in the theatre space should take a different function of "physical share" which cannot be "captured and written down" in the language of words. In Artaud's words, language functions in theatre as hieroglyphic writing in which "phonetic elements are coordinated to visual, pictorial and plastic elements." Derrida offers two arguments in terms of his reading of Artaud:

1. Derrida does not disagree with most of Artaud's ideas about the language of the stage. Instead, he disagrees when Artaud argues for a "pure presence" in theatre. Derrida considers "pure presence" a conceptual error on Artaud's part. As Derrida clarifies, *Artaud wanted to erase repetition*: he wants theatre to be in its "first time" of original movements, gestures and sounds without repeating it in the "second time" in order to make any meaning of its own. Rather he wants theatre to be the spectacle of experience of its own. Derrida argues that without repetition there is no identity, and "truth" can always be repeated "Repetition gathers and maintains the past-present as truth" through which identity is generated. What Derrida argues here is that human cognition operates by mediating the faculty of memory and the temporal phenomenon of repetition

without which there will not be any sense either to the world or to the Self. In this sense, Derrida suggests that while prophesying a spectacle of the "first time" Artaud envisaged a closed space outside of representation which also declares the Death of meaning.

2. *Artaud consumes a pure presence*, which means that Artaud does not want to preserve and maintain *present* as the manifestation of memory to be conscious of its presence. Rather, what he wants to do with theatre is Being with the *pure différance*, the difference which does not repeat. Derrida says that this *pure différance* is a reduced space of nowhere. 'Pure' is something which cannot be repeated and there will not be a meaning without a repetition. This is Derrida's criticism of Artaud: he declares the closure of representation by conceiving a 'place' outside the signifying process. As I shall demonstrate in Chapter four, here Derrida is addressing the issues of higher levels of consciousness by using the vocabulary from a different philosophical tradition.

What Derrida wants to say about the limitation of Artaud's theatre is that it does not *restore* the past and infuses it into present moment as a *trace*: it does not *restore* meaning or human behavioural patterns to re-cognize them as a repetition. Therefore, theatre of cruelty, for Derrida is the "art of difference" without "reserve" and without "return". It is a theatre "without history." Artaud wants to "repeat the proximity of *origin*" but only once. He also wants to save the "purity of a presence" without repetition.

Derrida's project focuses on a linguistic and historical context in which the signs *play* and repeat endlessly within the structure in order to make the sense of the presence of meaning possible. In contrast, Artaud rejects any kind of linguistic and historic structure of repetition particularly in theatre, arguing that "theatre is passionate overflowing, a frightful transfer of forces from body to body."[63] This *transfer of time* for Artaud does not seek a recognizable structure to *repeat*; rather it rests in motion, in time with gestures. In this sense, Artaud suggests a place outside the linguistic and historic time where the repetition repeats itself without reference and within the infinite. Derrida argues that there is no 'place' outside the linguistic and historic time and the place Artaud was suggesting is the *playing space* "of the world as play" and this play of life is artistic. At this point Derrida refers to two kinds of repetitions: 1) the repetition that indicates a movement back and forth and 2) the repetition that repeats itself as *original* without reference, which begins with its own representation. Derrida suggests that Artaud proposed a repetition without reference. Derrida's first category, repetition with movement refers to linguistic and historic time whereas repetition without reference is a state 'beyond' the linguistic and historic levels of meaning. As Derrida says, Artaud suggests the existence of a higher level of consciousness in performance by referring to a kind of repetition which repeats itself as *original*. In this repetition without reference, representation continues but not on historic or linguistic levels. The question left unanswered by Derrida is what the nature of that non-referential representation is and how a person can be aware of the existence of that level of non-historic and non-linguistic consciousness.

Derrida also did not address Artaud's views on breathing that he encountered with Balinese rituals. Artaud seems to have answers to both questions: actors' breathing and the non-referential repetition are interconnected, particularly with his view of theatre as the "frightful transfer of forces from body to body". Artaud refers to the functioning of different patterns of breathing helping to transfer the psycho-physical forces from body to body. Artaud combines these patterns of breathing and the actor's consciousness considering a different kind of performative working internally within the body.

Artaud, finding himself in the grey area of representation and the physical body, argued that meaning is brought about by our conceptual relations to objects, and whenever we intend to question this "object relationship" between meaning and form the result will be a total "chaos". What Artaud proposed is an "active language" for theatre, active in terms of exploring the actor's physical body and anarchic in terms of rejecting the psycho-linguistic representation, where "the usual limits of feeling and words are transcended."[64] A theatrical performance is always this *altered meaning* for Artaud, which he called *active metaphysics*, "the metaphysics [of body] out of language" that exists in relation to "time and movement." According to Artaud, theatre by its nature and definition is "destined to represent" but this does not mean that theatre could only represent human psychological conditions. For him, the true spirit of theatre allows understanding and experiencing "the known or unknown fields of consciousness,"[65] Artaud suggests breath as the new means for his new theatre in order to explore the "overflowing" of the "frightful transfer of forces" from body to body and from body to its unknown fields of consciousness. In different terms, Joseph R. Roach articulates the same idea by arguing that "beyond his rejection of literary texts, which supposedly doom the theatre to derivation, Artaud rooted his version of the paradox in the actor's breathing."[66]

No emotion is possible without a bodily localization corresponding to it. All human emotions are physically connected to the movements of the body. Human emotions, in this sense, are the result of complex movements linking both psychological and physical movements in the body. No movement is possible without its parallel breathing and therefore, each movement and each emotion of the body is theoretically interconnected.

While explaining a specific example, Cabbalistic theory and the practice of breathing, Artaud further asserts that "every mental movement, every feeling, every leap in human affectivity has an appropriate breath."[67] Artaud insists that the actor should depend on "the whetted edge of his breathing." However, this language remains vague and does not help us to understand fully the 'real' nature of the dynamics of breath in terms of physical force, emotion and its visual representation. Artaud, therefore, explains nothing of this natural property of the body, breath, except giving some vague ideas relating to different patterns of breathing, rhythm and sounds. However, he argues often strongly and clearly that the dynamics of breath is the power of the body and it can easily create memorable effects on thoughts and feelings including exploring the unknown fields of consciousness.

The following insights can be derived from the above sections evaluating performance and epistemological categories of performativity:

1. In the context of theatrical performance, performativity is a cognitive and emotional movement taking place in *between* the presented actions and their perception. The *embodied actions* as well as the *act of perception* are activities relating to the body and therefore, the body as an embodiment of psycho-physical elements in time and space functions as the basis of performativity. This means that both the *embodied actions* and the *act of perception* are the *movements* in time and space and therefore, performativity is a temporal element that operates within a performance situation between action and its reactions.

2. In the contexts of linguistics and philosophy, performativity is a conceptual movement involving temporisation of the field of the unconscious in terms of *presence* and its memory of the past. This means that the process of being aware of one's own being is a process in time where the self is positioned among other objects of signification. Thinkers like Nietzsche, Heidegger, Foucault, Deleuze and Derrida intend to make sense of this temporal element of meaning/consciousness from their own disciplines by using performance concepts and ideas.

3. Heidegger's *Wiederholung,* Deleuze's *repetition,* Foucault's *event* and Derrida's *différance* are epistemological concepts introducing the element of *time* in the production and reception of meaning. They all are referring to performativity by using different terms.

4. Artaud, through his idea of performativity, suggests a kind of 'repetition without reference' which he further connects with consciousness and actor's breathing.

5. Performativity, therefore, is explained in both the performance as well as in the epistemological categories as a psycho-physical movement involved in the production and reception of meaning.

All these views of performativity share a common idea that the appearance and disappearance of signs, objects and the body in time and space, mediated by perception, are the elements from which meaning emerges. Performativity, in all cases, is the dynamics of a psycho-physical movement which links past-present into a context of meaning that appears as a structure of signification. Performativity thus is a *play* between the Self and the structure of signification mediated by *time* that eventually leads towards identification; but this identification is never stabilized because of the passage of time: one cannot perceive an object similarly the second time around simply because the act of perception as well as the object of perception are temporal and that means, ever-changing. This process generates history for each appearance in space through the mediation of memory: it is a never-ending process and there is no space outside of this chain of signification. In short, performativity, in its nature and function, is this process of the production and reception of linguistic, aesthetic, social and philosophical representation of meanings.

Artaud accepts that representation is inevitable in theatre, but he intends to go beyond its chain of significations. Performativity, for him, is a temporal element of physical movement that reinforces the theatrical performance by the dynamics of breath. This means that Artaud's performativity is not related to the innermost characteristics of representation. For instance, when Deleuze classifies theatre as theatre of representation and theatre of repetition, he introduces movement to *mimesis* by arguing that the theatre of repetition is the temporal dimension of representation whereas the classical notion of representation is pictorial without movement. This means that even in Deleuze's repetition, the representational element is predominantly active. Only in the case of Artaud can we see the rejection of representation and the rediscovery of the "magic of breathing" in terms of an *active poetics* of theatre. When most of the thinkers of Artaud's time introduce movement in philosophy and poetics as *repetition* Artaud did separate repetition from re-presentation by conceiving a different notion of performativity, which is physical and non-conceptual. Inspired by a brief encounter with Balinese rituals and performance traditions, myths and beliefs, Artaud formulates a new means by which an actor can experience higher levels of consciousness. This new means, for Artaud, is breath. In order to establish the epistemological links between breath and consciousness, I will look at specific aspects of breath presented in the current philosophical thinking of Heidegger, Derrida and Irigaray.

1.4 Being and/or Breathing: Heidegger and Irigaray

Heidegger considered the issues of *Being* as the most specialized epistemological and metaphysical problem to be resolved: "why are there *essents* rather than nothing?"[68] The question why there is anything rather than nothing, for Heidegger is the first of all questions because it is the fundamental issue relating to our sense of Being. It is the fundamental issue because there is a passage of *time* in between the things *there* and *Being*. In *An Introduction to Metaphysics*, while explaining the fundamental nature of individual consciousness in relation to time and presence, Heidegger asks this question:

> And what is the temporal extension of human life amid all the millions of years? Scarcely a move of the second hand, a breath.

Was Heidegger aware of the role of breathing? Was he aware of the fact that breath functions as the physical base of the epistemological understanding of Being? Furthermore, this instance could be a metaphorical example of another truth: that the presence of Heidegger's thinking is activated and reinforced by an invisible *other*, his breathing. However, Heidegger says that breath is the "temporal extension" of our being and we ourselves "happen to belong" on this edge, the edge of breathing. If breath is considered as the temporal extension of being, is there a 'Being' without breathing? Luce Irigaray, in response to Heidegger's "forgetting of being," asks this fundamental question in her seminal book, *The Forgetting of Air in Martin Heidegger* as her fundamental rereading of Western metaphysics. In this, she offers a reassessment of *Air*, arguing that it is an all-persistent circulation of the material and the transcendental. In his essay, *The End of Philosophy and the Task of Thinking*, Heidegger asks some key questions in relation to his investigation of the proper matter for thinking by asking "in what circle are we here, and truly with no way out?"[69] That circle, for Heidegger is the circle of signifiers. Irigaray's rereading of Heidegger starts from this question and she asserts that there is also an unthinkable element within this circle of signifiers, the circle of *Air*. As she puts it: "of what [is] this *is*? Of air."[70]

Irigaray is skeptical about the entire formulation of the Western philosophical framework developed over centuries centred on and around the act of thinking, stating that "no wonder philosophy dies-without air."[71] She criticises the philosophers of Being, including Heidegger, of the *void* that they have created "by using up the air for telling without ever telling of air itself,"[72] For Irigaray, this is the chasm at the origin of their thought: "Can man live elsewhere than in air,"? Irigaray suggests that no habitation is possible neither in fire nor in water nor in the earth without air. The element of air is irreducibly constitutive to the human faculty of perception and the knowledge to re-cognize it. Air is always there, although we tend to forget it. It is an unrecognized "place of all presence and absence" and "no presence is possible without air". Irigaray talks about breath specifically, and for her, air is breath and the place of no breath is the place of disappearance. It plays between presence and absence, between life and death, between significations and their perception and between representation and its experience. This imperceptible materiality of air is the "forgotten *material mediation* of the *logos.*" Irigaray suggests that the air element is the mediation of all reflections including perception, language, thoughts, imagination and the faculty of action. In the particular context of signification and meaning, Irigaray asserts that air is the invisible *other*, which is irreducible and without which there is no movement between perception and cognition. We are in a space that is already occupied by air: two things cannot take place in the same place elsewhere other than the place of air.

Air is manifested as breath and for Irigaray, breath is a philosophical proposition against man's philosophy of "Being as the Being of forgetting" and as she suggests, the philosophy of breathing is the philosophy of living, a feminine act of "remembering." This philosophy is the philosophy of the *other*: the breath as the other of Being. Breath is the very act that links past-present and breathing is the present infinitive in which "future [turns down into] present". Breathing is the passage of time and the producer of consciousness.

Irigaray seems to be taking breath into the core of her philosophical thinking by saying that:

> Breathing corresponds to the first autonomous gesture of the living human being. To come into the world supposes inhaling and exhaling by oneself. In the uterus, we receive oxygen through the mother's blood. We are not yet autonomous, not yet born.[73]

Irigaray links breath to consciousness through the idea of autonomous entity of individual being. Breath for her is fundamental to all human activities including birth and death, and thoughts and actions. Further more, breathing in conscious for Irigaray, means taking care of one's life. Inspired by the classical texts of *Yoga*, Irigaray says "we are divided between two breaths, *the natural breath* and *the cultural breath…*"[74] The *natural breath* is the corporeal breathing and *the cultural breath* is the breathing, which is cultivated that is the spiritual breathing. As Irigaray further says, "…becoming spiritual means transforming our elemental vital breath little by little into a more subtle breath"[75] transcending corporeal breath into spiritual breath. Irigaray seems to be referring to a practice of breathing, based on *Yoga*, by saying that breath combines human consciousness and physical body. But, it is not clear from her writings that what kind of practice does she referring to. However, the equation of breathing is *Being* is clearly established in Irigaray as air is the form of "inspiration" manifests in exercising the physical movements of the body, including perception and its re-cognition. Irigaray locates breath epistemologically in performativity.

Summary

To conclude, this chapter intends to identify the epistemological location of breath in a wider context of performativity as a process of perception and meaning. While investigating the nature of performativity in the contexts of theatrical performance as well as critical theory, the following points can be summarized:

1. Performativity is a temporal concept explaining the nature of the production and reception of meaning by incorporating body, signs, language and the field of human sub-conscious as its basic elements.

2. Performativity, from a theatrical performance perspective, is a process linking physical performance and its reception into meaning and emotional experience.

3. In a critical discourse, performativity is again explained as an epistemological process linking *past-present* through a psycho-physical movement of *repetition* within the field of significations in order to produce meaning, history and consciousness.

4. The presence of the body as the *presence* and its *perception* are the basis for the functioning of performativity in various linguistic, cultural and social contexts.

5. Performativity, for Artaud, is the dynamics of actor's breathing, linking consciousness and the physical body in a performance. Ritual elements of performance and breathing patterns form the basis of Artaud's theatricality.

6. Irigaray's idea of performativity is located in breath in the following manner:

    a. Air is the fundamental element and the only place where all the mental and physical activities of human beings are taking place.
    b. It is the invisible *other* that produces meaning and forms of representations of poetry and thoughts.
    c. Without the materiality of air, there is no representation of thought or art and there is no exercising of physical movements, perception and therefore, no cognition.

The flow of breath is the flow of *presence* and *absence* and therefore, the flow of breath is the flow of meaning. Breathing is a movement that connects physical and mental activities together and therefore, it is a movement of action, meaning and experience. The flow of breath is the passage of *time* that brings words, movements of the body, human actions and thoughts into contact with each other in its place. Breath also reinforces the fields of known and unknown levels of consciousness. As breath is physically located in the body, it is also located, epistemologically, in the functioning of performativity as a process of production and reception of meaning. In other words, as I propose in the chapter, the materiality of *breath* is located as an essential element in the process of meaning and consciousness within the structure of significations. This physical material, breath, located epistemologically in performativity also suggests the transformational borders between known and unknown fields of consciousness (I will look at this aspect in the fourth Chapter in details). Therefore, breath is *bio-theatricality* and the *invisible Other* that reinforce meaning into performativity. In the following chapter, I investigate how breath is understood, explained and practiced in the traditional cultures, searching for a working methodology and system of knowledge useful to contemporary theatre practice and consciousness studies.

Notes

[1] Tracy C Davis and Thomas Postlewait, ed. *Theatricality*, (Cambridge: Cambridge University Press, 2003), pp. 2-39.
[2] Ibid., p. 6.
[3] Ibid., pp. 4 -7.
[4] King, ct. in Ibid., p. 5.
[5] Sara Grant, *Sankaracarya's Concept of Relation,* (New Delhi: Motilal Banarsidass, 1999), p. 19.
[6] Willmar Sauter, *The Theatrical Event: Dynamics of Performance and Perception*, (Iowa City: University of Iowa Press, 2000), pp. 50-3.
[7] Ibid., p. 50.
[8] Roland Barthes, ct. in Tracy C Davis and Thomas Postlewait, ed. *Theatricality*, (Cambridge: Cambridge University Press, 2003), p. 23.
[9] Ibid., p. 24.
[10] Erika Fischer-Lichte, " Theatricality", in *Theatre Research International* (TRI) 20.2. 1997: pp. 218-60.
[11] Tracy C Davis and Thomas Postlewait, ed. *Theatricality*, (Cambridge: Cambridge University Press, 2003), p. 27.
[12] Josette Féral, ct. in. Ibid., p. 27.
[13] Paul de Man, *Allegories of Reading: Figural Language in Rousseau, Nietzsche, Rilke and Proust* (New Haven, 1979) p. 298.
[14] Peggy Phelan, *Unmarked: the Politics of Performance*, (London & New York: Routledge, 1993), pp. 146-49.
[15] Ibid., p. 146.
[16] Richard Schechner, *Performance Studies: An Introduction,* (London & New York: Routledge, 2002), p. 110.
[17] Willmar Sauter, *The Theatrical Event: Dynamics of Performance and Perception*, (Iowa City: University of Iowa Press, 2000), p. 56.
[18] Marvin Carlson, *Theatre Research International*, (TRI) 20.2. 1996: pp. 100-120.
[19] Erika Fischer-Lichte, "Theatricality", in *Theatre Research International* 20.2. 1997: pp. 218-260.
[20] Ibid., p. 52
[21] Ibid., p. 52.
[22] Ibid., pp. 54-6.
[23] Willmar Sauter, "Who Is Who and What Is What? Introductory Notes," in *Advances in Reception and Audience Research,* vol.2, pp. 5-16.
[24] Nicola Frijda, cited in Willmar Sauter, *The Theatrical Event: Dynamics of Performance and Perception*, (Iowa City: University of Iowa Press, 2000), p. 58.
[25] Ibid., p. 59.
[26] Ibid., p. 63.
[27] Ibid,. pp. 62-3.
[28] William H. Ittelson, *Visual Space Perception,* (New York: Springer Publishing Company, 1960), pp. 5-6.
[29] Ibid., p. 6.
[30] Daniel Meyer Dinkgräfe, (1999) 'Consciousness and the Concept of Rasa', *Performing Arts Journal,* vol.1, part 4, pp. 103-115.

[31] Willmar Sauter, *The Theatrical Event: Dynamics of Performance and Perception*, (Iowa City: University of Iowa Press, 2000), p. 70.
[32] Michel Foucault, "*Theatrum Philosophicum*", in Timothy Murray, ed. *Mimesis, Masochism and Mime: The Politics of Theatricality in Contemporary French Thought,* (Ann Arbor: Michigan University Press, 1997) pp. 222-223.
[33] Ibid., p. 223.
[34] Ibid., p. 223.
[35] Ibid., p. 223.
[36] Ibid., p. 223.
[37] Ibid., p. 223.
[38] Paul Patton, *Deleuze and the Political,* (London: Routledge, 2000), pp. 27-8.
[39] Michael Foucault, "Theatrum Philosophicum" c.f. Timothy Murray, (ed). *Mimesis, Masochism and Mime: The politics of Theatricality in Contemporary French Thought,* (Ann Arbor: University of Michigan Press, 1997), p. 222.
[40] Gilles Deleuze, *The Logic of Sense*, tr. Mark Lester, with Charles Stivale, ed. Constantin V. Boundas, (New York: Columbia University Press, 1990), p. 63.
[41] Martin Heidegger, *Nietzsche* (Pfullingen: Neste, 1961), vol. p. 215, ct. in Arne Melberg, *Theories of Mimesis*, (Cambridge: Cambridge University Press, 1995), pp. 3-4.
[42] Ibid., p. 4.
[43] Ibid., p. 1.
[44] <http://plato.stanford.edu/entries/descartes-epistemology/#4> (consulted March 12, 2005).
[45] Gilles Deleuze, *Difference and Repetition,* (London& New York: Continuum, 2001), p. 8.
[46] Ibid., p. 8
[47] Ibid., p. 10.
[48] Gilles Deleuze, *Difference and Repetition,* (London& New York: Continuum, 2001), p. 10.
[49] Ibid., p. 10.
[50] Ibid., p. 10.
[51] Ibid., p. 13.
[52] Jacques Derrida, *Margins of Philosophy*, tr. Alan Bass, (Chicago: The University of Chicago Press, 1982), pp. 3-9.
[53] Martin Heidegger, *Sein und Zeit,* (Tübingen: Niemeyer, 1986) ct. in Arne Melberg, *Theories of Mimesis*, (Cambridge: Cambridge University Press, 1995),pp. 154-59.
[54] Ibid., p. 155.
[55] Ibid., p. 157.
[56] Jacques Derrida, "Signature Event Context" in *Margins of Philosophy*, tr. Alan Bass, (Chicago: The University of Chicago Press, 1982), p. 315.
[57] Jacques Derrida, "Différance" in *Margins of Philosophy*, tr. Alan Bass, (Chicago: The University of Chicago Press, 1982), p. 7.
[58] See for more details on this in Ibid., pp. 18-22.
[59] Claude Schumacher with Brian Singleton, (ed.) *Artaud on Theatre*, (London: Methuen, 2001), p. 119. I follow this edition only for one letter which is missing Victor Corti's English translation of *Theatre and Its Double* (1970). But, I largely follow Victor Corti because the original text is more or less unedited in Corti where as

in Schumacher and Singleton, many crucial portions have been omitted. For instance, in their 2001 edition, Artaud's classification of various patterns of breathing is missing (p. 141), which is more important to this thesis.
[60] Ibid., p. 80.
[61] Jacques Derrida, "The Theatre of Cruelty and the Closure of Representation" in Timothy Murray, ed. *Mimesis, Masochism and Mime: The Politics of Theatricality in Contemporary French Thought,* (Ann Arbor: Michigan University Press, 1997), p. 42.
[62] Ibid., p. 46.
[63] Ibid., p. 59.
[64] Antonin Artaud, *Theatre and Its Double*, tr. Victor Corti, (London: Calder & Boyars, 1970), p. 30.
[65] Ibid., p. 35.
[66] Joseph R. Roach, *The Player's Passion: Studies in the Science of Acting,* (Ann Arbor: University of Michigan Press, 1999), p. 223.
[67] Ibid., p. 89.
[68] Martin Heidegger, *An Introduction to Metaphysics*, tr. Ralph Manheim, (New Delhi: Motilal Banarsidass, 1999), p. 1. The word *essents* stands for existence or things that are, which according to the translator, is coined by himself because the original German word *Dasein* refers to an every day meaning of 'existence'. But, when Heidegger uses this word in his philosophical writings, he splits the word as *Da-sein,* meaning being-there. So, according to the translator's opinion, *essents* is the most nearest word in English that expresses the very meaning. In my view, there is a time element in between the split words of *Da-sein* in Heidegger which is not at a concern of the translator. However, I use this word *essent* since I follow this edition.
[69] Martin Heidegger, "The End of Philosophy and the Task of Thinking" in *Basic Writings*, tr. David Farrell Krell, (New York: Harper Collins, 1993), p. 449.
[70] Luce Irigaray, *The Forgetting of Air*, tr. Mary Beth Mader, (London: Athlone Press, 1999), p. 5.
[71] Ibid., p. 5.
[72] Ibid., p. 7.
[73] Luce Irigaray, *Between East and West,* (New York: Columbia University Press, 2002), p. 73
[74] Ibid., p. 75.
[75] Ibid., p. 76.

Chapter Two
In Search of Breath

Breath is located in the body and serves as the basis of theatricality in everyday life, through combining speech, action and thoughts in relation to an explicit level of meaning. The psycho-physicality of human embodiment is activated through the act of breathing. Breath as the fundamental source of energy to all human actions, reactions, emotions and speech, is an inseparable element in the nature of human embodiment. The movement of the breath is the movement of the body and the flow of breath is the flow of language and therefore, meaning. All the body's physical, mental and linguistic activities are deeply interconnected with the dynamics of breath in the body. Many of the cultural, religious, mythical and philosophical traditions of the world possess, in one way or another, some forms of knowledge related to the importance of breathing. Aristotle's *On Breath*, for instance, investigates the physiological and metaphysical functioning of breath in the body while examining pre-existent views of the ways in which breath has been conceived of and debated in the Greek natural philosophical tradition since Diogenes and Democritus. Aristotle elaborates these initial observations of the functioning of breath in the body further in his metaphysical speculations, arguing that the Soul and emotions are interconnected with the dynamics of breath.

The linguistic derivations of breath-related words in various languages suggest different understandings of the implications of the concepts and practices of breath. The word spirit, for instance, comes from the Latin word *spiritus*, which literally means breath. Although the Sanskrit word *prana* and the Tamil word *uyir* continue to have multiple levels of meaning, the initial meaning of the word *prana* in Sanskrit is *soul*. There are several other words in Sanskrit derived from *prana* that refer to some forms of breath-related practice or activity, such as *pranakarmani* which means the functions of life breath, *pranam* which means the air that acts outwardly, *pranavayu* which means the vital air that moves in the chest, and *pranapanu*, which refers to air moving up and down. Similarly, in the Tamil language, the word *uyir* refers to meanings such as soul, ascendant, one of the vital airs, wind, voice and spoken sound. The word *uyir-ttal* in Tamil literally means "to regain consciousness". The breath-related words in Sanskrit and Tamil imply the existence of specific practices and philosophies related to breath. The South Indian Shiva tradition, a sub-category of Tamil, for instance, offers a systematic approach to breathing through various systems of practice like *Siddha Yoga*, martial arts and medicine, which are interconnected with each other in terms of their specific references to breath.

2.1. Aristotle and Breath

Some pre-Aristotelian natural philosophers of Greece, including Diogenes and Democritus had dealt with respiration and some of them had offered no explanations at all. Others had discussed it without much insight and without sufficient experience of the facts. Aristotle, therefore, began to address questions related to respiration in *Prava Naturalia*. The book includes two treatises on breath: *On Respiration* and *On Breath.*[1]

In today's Aristotle scholarship, the authorship of these treatises is under question. Hett's views on this debate as follows: First, the writer of the treatises confuses the reader's understanding of natural human respiration by mentioning a 'connatural breathing'. It is not clear in the treatises whether the writer is here referring to some pattern or technique of breathing in human respiration known only to him. According to Hett, the writer never explains clearly what he understands by this 'connatural breathing', but obviously it is not the same thing as ordinary breath. The second argument is that the writer makes constant use of the word 'air-duct' in *On Breath*, which applies primarily to windpipe (481 a 22, b 13 & 484 a 14).[2] As Hett argues, the writer uses the word with no reference to any 'duct' again in *On Breath*, which apparently refers to the arteries.[3] The treatises, *On Breath* and *On Respiration*, thus lack the consistency and clarity characteristic of texts where Aristotle's authorship is not in dispute.

The texts do, however, establish physiological links between air and nutriment by saying that "the veins and air ducts…are probably the vehicles of nutriment."[4] These veins and air ducts are connected with the intestines and the belly. Similarly, the texts demonstrate the link between emotions and breath when discussing pulsation. In this sense, the writer's understanding of the physiological and psychological functioning of breath in the body is worth considering. Rather than addressing the historical questions of authorship here, I would like to assume the text is by Aristotle, if only for the sake of convenience, and summarise the key concepts illustrated by Aristotle on breath and its relation to the human body and consciousness. Bearing in mind the criticisms that Aristotle made obvious mistakes in understanding human physiology and its system of breathing, I am still interested in looking at whether he makes some sense in his attempt to establish the link between breath, consciousness and emotion in the human embodiment.

In his discussion of breath, Aristotle is concerned with two questions: why some living creatures are long-lived and others short-lived. He also raises the questions of whether the length of a life-span is necessarily related to the state of the human organism's health, and what the element common to natural objects is that renders them open to be easily destroyed. The latter question derives from Aristotle's observation that knowledge, health and disease have their own peculiar form of destruction. For instance, learning and recollection destroy ignorance, whereas forgetfulness and error destroy knowledge. Furthermore, knowledge can be destroyed even when the human organism that contains them is not destroyed. However, when the structure of the natural object, the human organism, is destroyed, the knowledge or health that is in them are also destroyed. As a result of these insights, Aristotle was interested in examining the inner truths of the combinations of the natural elements in the human organism. In his ontology of being and destruction it would be impossible for anything that has no opposite to be destroyed. In other words, only opposites are destroyed, for everything which possesses matter must have an opposite in some sense. Ultimately, then, every form of matter is destroyed by its environment through a process of movement in which the form is either being created or destroyed. For instance, the lesser flame is consumed by the greater flame because the nourishment, the smoke, is exhausted rapidly by the greater. Aristotle compares all kinds of growth and destruction with movement saying that "everything is in a state of movement, and is being either generated or destroyed."[5] The longevity of creatures, in this context, is a dynamic efficacy belonging to both space and time, mediated by movement. Aristotle developed this concept of spatio-temporal movement further in relation to *air*, drawing on observable facts, for example, that the dead body is cold and dry whereas the living body is moist and warm. From this observation he concluded that the matter of which all things are composed consists of hot and cold, dry and moist. Thus, the difference between the cold and dry dead body and the warm and moist living body, according to Aristotle, is that one contains the *air* element that the other does not contain. I will further develop this theme of the inter-connectedness of breath, movement and time in Chapter Four in relation to the Siddha *Yoga* mode of physical philosophy and the extended levels of consciousness known as *Savikalpa Samadhi* and *Nirvikalpa Samadhi,* because, according to Siddha *Yoga*, breath as a movement indicates time and further links the body and consciousness. The following sections will briefly illustrate Aristotle's key themes on breath.

2.1.1 Breath is a Body

In a close observation of the functioning of breath, Aristotle says that nutriment is the element which animates the body and therefore we have to consider the nature and source of nutriment in terms of breath. Nutrition may occur in two ways: by respiration and by digestion of food. Breath is a nutriment to the body in the same way that food is. For Aristotle, breath thus has a material nature, just as food has. Aristotle clearly specifies the distinct but related functions in the body of breath / air and food: breath / air is the agent that produces activity by employing the digestive faculty that in turn causes growth and nourishment. Going into detail about the functions of breath, understood as "the purest substance of the body,"[6] within the overall functioning of the body, Aristotle argues that breathing serves the purpose of refrigeration: by drawing cool air in, heat is cooled down. There are three distinct movements of breath: respiration, pulsation and the action upon food. The movements of pulsation and respiration are perceptible to a certain extent, whereas "the movement that affects nutriment is almost theoretical, but, in so far as it can be determined from its result, it is a matter of perception" (*On Breath*, IV:497). Aristotle argues that nutritive movement is the result of respiration and that this movement will not be uniform throughout the body. Pulsation is relatively distinct from the other two. The cause of pulsation is “the trapping of the air within” (*On Breath*, IV: 497); it is primary and has its own origin, which is found initially in the heart and from here it is communicated to the other organs. At this point Aristotle clearly describes pulsation as the “…animal’s underlying essence, which is realized in activity” (*On Breath*, IV: 497). The word ‘animal’ refers to all breathing animals including humans. Aristotle’s attempt here is to establish the link between bodily activities and pulsation as an underlying essence of animal activity, and therefore, he takes his argument further into the discussion of the origin of pulsation.

Of the three functions of breath in the body, pulsation and respiration are prior in origin and pulsation in turn is prior to respiration. As Aristotle explains the mechanism, respiration starts as soon as the embryo is released from the womb “and ingestion and nutrition belong to it both during and after its formation, but pulsation begins at the very outset, while the heart is forming, as can be observed in eggs. So that pulsation is prior in origin, and resembles an activity, and not an interception of breath, except in so far as this contributes to its activity” (*On Breath*, IV: 499). Aristotle argues that pulsation is the first movement or the first act of animation that is perceptible and the foremost indication of life in the embryo, even before the first breath takes place in the human organism. Breath, for Aristotle, contributes to the growth and animation of the human body through the physical activity of respiration. The terms breath and respiration need clarification here, though the distinction is not clear in Aristotle: breath is the substance and respiration is the process in which the substance nourishes the organism. Aristotle’s observation of breath as the underlying essence of human activity is crucial to the major argument in the thesis that says that breath as a voluntary human action influences states and levels of consciousness.

2.1.2 Breath and Soul

In relation to the idea of pulsation as underlying animal activity, Aristotle further examines the connection between breathing and pulsation in relation to the psychological conditions of the mind. Following his own earlier observation of pulsation as “the trapping of the air within [the body] Aristotle asks another question why breath gets attracted and trapped perpetually within, for no apparent external reasons. The perpetually repeating cycles of inhalation and exhalation, for Aristotle, seem to be the trapping of air within the body. Aristotle describes the origin of breath as having its source from within, either as a "function of the soul" or "soul itself or else some mixture of bodies which by their means cause this attraction" (*On Breath*, IV: 497). While thus linking breath and pulsation, Aristotle further asserts that breathing is a pulsation which is the primary act and 'the underlying essence of animals'. This means that, for Aristotle, pulsation, breath and soul are the fundamental principles interlinking the physical and the psychological experience of the body because movement and sensation are the two matching qualities through which the soul operates in the body (*On the Soul*: I. II: 29).[7] As he puts it:

> Those then who have interpreted the soul in terms of motion have regarded the soul as most capable of producing movement. But those who have referred it to cognition and perception regard the soul as the first beginning of all things- (*On the Soul*; I. II: 23).

Aristotle acknowledges that all the physical, physiological and intellectual faculties in a human organism are profound demonstrations of the interconnections between breath and its subsequent movements in the body. While considering movement, sensation and incorporeality as the three attributes of the soul, Aristotle places breath at the centre of his philosophical thinking as the basis of the formation of the soul: "breath is the purest substance of the body" (*On Breath*, I.II: 489). For Aristotle, the soul on the one hand represents the idea of human embodiment, which is the physical basis of all the human experiences of mind and body. On the other hand, the soul is explained as the appearance of breath in the body which causes the functioning of movement, sensation and mind. These views together elucidate the role of breath in understanding the nature of all the psycho-physical activities of human existence. Aristotle's this view of the psychological implications of breath further supports my arguments in the thesis establishing the links between breath and emotion.

2.1.3 Breath and Emotion

The link between breath and emotion (using the term synonymously, for the purposes of my argument, with affections and feelings) is clearly established in Aristotle when he discusses the possible entangling of pulsation and emotions. Irregularities in pulsation will occur "during conditions of fear, expectations and conflict" (*On Breath*, IV.V:499). Aristotle argues that in most cases, none of the emotions, whether active or passive, can exist apart from the body and this also applies to emotions like anger, courage, desire and sensation. Therefore:

> Probably all the affections of the soul are associated with the body—anger, gentleness, fear, pity, courage and joy, as well as loving and hating; for when they appear the body is also affected. (*On the Soul*, I.I: 15).

There are times when no irritation or fear is expressed although the provocations are strong and obvious. Similarly, small and obscure effects produce movement when the body is disposed to anger and when the person is in an angry mood. Interestingly, sometimes humans show all the symptoms of fear without any cause of fear being present. Hence, for Aristotle, emotions and "affections of the soul are formulae expressed in matter" (*On the Soul*, I.I: 15) and these must be defined as the movements of the body or of a part or faculty of the body. Considering the value of the argument that Aristotle establishes in terms of breath and its psycho-physical movements, it is obvious that each physical movement and each mental reflection must have a corresponding movement of breath in the body, linking physical activities and mental experiences together. For Aristotle, breath is the pure substance of the body that activates the process of respiration, and all the psycho-physical movements including emotions and physical animations are the results of the dynamics of breath in the body. As we could see, Aristotle's position regarding the interrelations between soul and the body is essentially dualist, which considers body and mind as two separate entities. But, it is also interesting to see the importance that Aristotle has given to breathing suggesting that breath is the key element that links mind and the body. Aristotle's idea of the soul, in this sense, is a metaphorical concept explaining the significance of the dynamics of breathing within the psycho-physicality of human existence. Aristotle's this view on breath is significantly important to my thesis because this psycho-physical foundation of breath as an autonomous human activity provides ground to my further arguments in Chapter four linking breath and consciousness in the background of Saivite philosophy in general and *Siddha Yoga* of South India in particular. In yogic philosophy, breath is the essential element which is underlying the basic nature of individual consciousness, and alterations on level of consciousness have connections to alterations on patterns of breathing. So, according to South Indian *Siddha yoga*, dualism in individual perception is a state of consciousness, which can be altered through appropriate alterations in daily breathing. In short, through the idea of the soul, Aristotle demonstrates breath as an essential element underpinning human consciousness. The same idea can be found in *Siddha yoga*, as a fully developed philosophical view and practice based on breath (See Chapter 4).

2.2 *Tao* and Breath

T'ai Ch'i Ch'uan is a Chinese martial arts form, perhaps the one that is most well-known in the West today, often under its abbreviated name *T'ai Ch'i.* The tradition has been ascribed to the thirteenth century Taoist priest, Chang Sang Feng, who began training the monks of Shaolin, situated upon the mountain of Wutang. Chang Sang Feng and his Taoist priests encouraged the development of various martial arts traditions in China. However, *T'ai Ch'i* flourished between the eighteenth and nineteenth centuries in China. Known as a system of self-defence, *T'ai Ch'i* opposes force by yielding and defeats external force with internal force. *Ch'i* is breath. It is the air that we breathe in order to sustain vitality and energy in the body. According to the explanations provided by the *T'ai Ch'i* system, *Ch'i* operates the bipolar dynamics of *Yin* and *Yang*: what we breathe in is *Yin* and what we breathe out is *Yang*. As Paul Wildish, a senior martial arts practitioner of *T'ai Ch'i* in the UK, puts it: "this bipolarity is the constant of the inner alchemy schema and is present in each aspect of the functions and movement of *Ch'i*."[8] *Ch'i* is said to be the primary energetic force from which the basic substance of all life and matter is formed, and it is activated through the interaction of *Yin* and *Yang*. As Wildish further explains these principles, *Ch'i*, as the basic substance, can exist without form and it can also exist in the form of a thought or action, the spiritual or material. The non-material states are pure energy, which is *Yang,* whereas the physical and material states are affiliated to *Yin.* According to the doctrines of Tao philosophy, establishing a natural cyclic equilibrium of these two forces is the strongest basis of good physical and mental health. In Taoist cosmology, there are three powers that govern the flow of *Ch'i*, which are Heaven, the *Yang*, Earth, the *Yin*, and Man, the *Yin* and *Yang*. The nature of the bipolar dynamic of *Ch'i* is explained by the claim that *Yang Ch'i* flows downward from Heaven, whereas Ying *Ch'i* follows upward from Earth and in the zone of man, which lies between them, these two flows meet and combine. The flow of these three elements of air in the body is considered as the Three Treasures of *Jing, Ch'i* and *Shen*: *Jing* is known as the essence, *Ch'i* is vital energy and *Shen* is the spirit. *Jing*, *Ch'i* and *Shen* are further considered as the fundamental essences of body, breath and mind; maintaining their relative strength and balance will result in the longevity and health of the human being.

Wildish points out that according to Tao philosophy and Chinese medicine, *Jing*, *Ch'i* and *Shen* are located at three elixir fields in the body. *Jing*, the primordial essence, is positioned in the lower elixir field, below the navel, and is associated with human sexual glands. *Ch'i* is located in the middle elixir field around the solar plexus and is linked to the adrenal glands. *Shen*, or spirit, is centred in the head and is related to the pituitary and pineal glands. As Wildish states, "the internal alchemy of Taoism transforms essence into energy, energy into spirit and sprit into the vital qualities of the universe, the mysterious resonance of power, compassion and wisdom."[9] Taoists believe that all creation is subject to the rule of the five elements of Wood, Fire, Earth, Metal and Water and these elements each have a season and a time of day when their influence is stronger in the body than that of the others. This five element theory is employed in Tao-based Chinese medicine as a principle to counteract imbalances by using the forces of one element to support or counteract the forces of or more of the other elements in order to restore the equilibrium of the body. These five elements of the body, and sensations and emotions, are closely connected to *Ch'i* and its flow in the meridian lines in the body.

2.2.1 *Ch'i* Meridians

Ch'i circulates all over the body along the meridian lines. A meridian line is understood as a pathway of energy that forms a close relationship with all the organs and the flow of blood in the body. Wildish explains that in the context of the nature and function of meridians, *Ch'i* is the energetic *Yang* force that moves blood around the body; blood is understood as the material form of *Ch'i*, nourishing the organs where *Ch'i* is generated. "As *Ch'i* moves the blood, the blood moves *Ch'i*."[10] This follows the principles of *Yin* and *Yang* in which each contains the element of the other. When the flow of *Ch'i* is blocked in the body, the affected organs will malfunction due to the slowing down of the blood flow. Thus, the approach of Tao-based Chinese medicine is applied as an intervention to unblock the meridian flow in the body.

There are twelve main meridians in the body: the *Yang* meridians are located on the back and the outside surface of the limbs, and the *Yin* meridians are located on the inner surface of the limbs and the front of the body. *Ch'i* flows downward through the *Yang* channels and upward through the *Yin* channels as opposing forces, maintaining balance in the body. In addition to these twelve meridians, there are eight other meridian channels running deeper beneath the surface of the body and these are known as the reservoirs of *Ch'i* that cross the twelve primary meridians at several locations in the body. These deeper circulating channels, according to Tao-based Chinese medicine, are the most important meridians in the body and are divided into two groups: the Governing Vessels and the Directing Vessels. These Vessels are located directly on the front and rear of the body. As Wildish explains, the Governing Vessels regulate all the *Yang* channels in the body while it runs up the spine from the bottom to the head, whereas the Directing Vessels regulate all the *Yin* channels while it runs up the front of the body over the stomach and chest to the throat and mouth. The flow of *Ch'i* all over the meridian channels maintains the overall health and the chemical balance of the body through the circulation of blood and other body fluids. Thus the most important aspect of Tao-based Chinese medical practice is the power of *Ch'i* or the breath.

2.2.2 *Ch'i Kung* and Breath

Ch'i Kung is a breath-related practice through which the two aspects of *Ch'i*, the *Yang* and *Yin*, are cultivated and maintained in the body by finding a proper harmony in human respiration. The term *Ch'i Kung* is used to describe a category of exercises, techniques and styles of the body and its energy dynamics. The origin of *Ch'i Kung* goes back to the practices of the shamans and ancient Taoist monks. So, *T'ai-Ch'i* and *Ch'i Kung* are two schools of practice based on breath developed from Tao-Buddhism. There are two forms available in this system of practice - still practice and moving practice; both conform to the dynamic of *Yang* and *Yin* in the body. Moving forms are those that involve the external exercise and movement of the body while keeping the mind still. Still forms encourage cultivating the internal movement of breath while keeping the body still. Both are practices of meditation and seek to co-ordinate breathing and bodily movements in rhythmic harmony. Still forms include meditation positions such as sitting on a chair, cross legged in the lotus-position and standing, while the moving forms encompass a broad range of exercises and movement techniques whose origin dates back to ancient Taoist monks. In both forms, still and moving, the practitioner is asked always to maintain the position of the spine in central alignment with the head in order to stimulate the flow of *Ch'i* from the lower abdomen to the head and vice versa.

In the description of both the still and the moving practices of *Ch'i Kung* found in Wildish, breath is the unifying element. The aim of these practices is to unblock the flow of *Ch'i* by co-ordinating movement and breath and stillness and breath. According to Wildish, *Ch'i Kung* offers techniques to strengthen the full capacity of the lungs and control and modulate breath in order to maximize energy; this is also the objective of Indian *Yoga*. All *Ch'i Kung* breathing exercises aim to increase the capacity of breath and conserve vital energy through the depth and frequency of inhalation and exhalation. The two most familiar breathing methods used in *Ch'i Kung* are: natural abdominal breathing and reverse abdominal breathing. Wildish describes them as follows:[11]

1. *Natural Abdominal Breathing:* this technique involves drawing air slowly and evenly in through the nostrils to the bottom of the lungs while the diaphragm is pressed downward to expand the abdomen. As the practitioner breathes out slowly, the abdomen is relaxed and drawn in. Between each cycle the body is relaxed and allowed to recover its natural posture.

2. *Reverse Abdominal Breathing:* this technique, as its name implies, is the opposite of the natural abdominal method. In this cycle, instead of expanding the stomach on inhalation, it is contracted and relaxed on exhalation.

Both these abdominal breathing methods stimulate and massage organs and glands and convert the diaphragm into a second heart, assisting circulation and the efficiency of the lungs. Other *Ch'i Kung* breathing techniques described by Wildish include vibratory sounds using the syllable 'ah' or mantras similar to *Yoga*. These resonating sounds vibrate in different zones of the body, thus enhancing the energy levels in those zones by strengthening *Ch'i*. Like Indian *Yoga*, *Ch'i Kung* identifies a centre in the body, which is located two inches below the navel in the lower elixir field. This point, in almost all the medical, spiritual and martial arts traditions of the East, represents the centre of the body's vital energy. This centre is also the centre of gravity of the body. This centre, which is called *Swātistāna* in Indian *trantric* and *yogic* tradition is also said to be the focal point where all the psycho-physical forces in the body are integrated and stored. Hence, breathing and movement techniques described in *Ch'i Kung*, *Yoga* and other similar practices are aimed at exploring the concealed form of energy within the body. Chinese martial and spiritual traditions are, historically, in many ways indebted to various Indian systems like *Tantra*, *Yoga* and martial arts. Unlike the Chinese systems, many of the Indian traditions like, Agastiya's *Marma Therapy* and South Indian *Siddha Yoga,* still seem to be unfamiliar to the world, in particular the West, mainly because of their antiquity and the degree of confidentiality maintained among their practitioners. Further to Aristotle, this section shows how breath has been developed as a systematic practice in Chinese traditions of martial arts and physiotherapy. The following observations can be listed as the summary of this section:

1. Breath is central to religion, philosophy, medicine and martial arts of China. *T'ai Ch'i*, as an example, shows a systematic physical approach, which is informed by breathing.

2. They are attempts to locate individual and cosmic links by establishing the connection between the body, breathing, physical animation and higher level of consciousness.

3. Breath is systematically employed in *Ch'i Kung* and other similar physical techniques like Indian *Tantra* and *Yoga* aiming to explore the psycho-physical energy level of the body. This fundamental approach to breath in relation to the psycho-physical energy level of the body is the basic method found in many systems of actor training available in some of the traditional performance forms like *Kathakali*, *Kudiyattam* and *Noh*.

4. The approach to theatricality, therefore, in these traditions are informed by the ways in which breath is used in terms of the physical, psychological and consciousness levels of the actor's art. I will look at this aspect in Chapter 3, in the context of *Kudiyattam* and Sanskrit tradition (sections 3.1, 3.1.1, 3.1.2 & 3.1. 3) and *Noh* in contemporary actor training (section 3.1.4.).

The insights gained from this section pave the way to allow a deeper understanding of how breath has been understood, presented and practiced in various Indian traditions of philosophy, spirituality and other physical practices like medicine and physiotherapy.

2.3 Breath and the Sanskrit Tradition

The concept of *Prana,* breath, is not only central to Indian philosophical thinking but also acts as a fundamental source to form the basis of various practices like medicine, martial arts and performance. The theoretical and practical aspects of *Prana* are discussed systematically and elaborately in various systems of knowledge in the Sanskrit tradition as a material phenomenon, which explains in depth our understanding of the conditions of linguistic meaning, visibility, appearance, human actions, voice and altered levels of consciousness. The *Sāmkhya* philosophical system, which is considered as one of the major influences in post-Vedic Indian thought and which is also constantly referred to in different stages of Sanskrit literature, deserves special attention in this context. Concerning the systematic implications of the *Sāmkhya* doctrine of the "accumulation theory" of derivation,[12] the subtle sound element (*śabdatanmātra*) generates the gross element of *ākāśa*, space; the subtle touch element (*sparśatanmātra*), combined with the subtle sound element, generates the gross element of *vāyu*, air. *Prana* is the dynamic force of air present in the body as a vital force, which motivates human respiration. *Akasa,* space, includes v*āyu*, air. There are two kinds of space according to *Sāmkhya*: the universal outer space and the inner space of consciousness. According to Wilhelm Halbfass, the *Chāndogya Upanishad*, (VIII, 1, 3) states: "As far as this world – space (*ayam – akasah)* extends, so far extends the space within the inner "heart" (*antarhrdaya – ākāsah*)."[13] The word 'heart' here does not carry any anatomical meaning as the hollow muscular organ that pumps the blood throughout the body. Rather, the word suggests a spatial dimension in human consciousness. The 'heart' as an abode or seat of consciousness in the body is a well recognised idea proposed by some schools of thought of Indian philosophy. As it is suggested in the *Upanisad*, within these two spaces are contained both heaven and earth, both fire and wind, both sun and moon, lighting and stars, both that which is available to somebody in this world and that which is not – all that is contained in it (*sarvam tad asmin samāhitam*). In the same *Upanishad*, the hymnic teaching of Sāndilya says that the self is "of the nature of space" (*ākāsātman*). As Halbfass further explains, the correlation and concordance between external space and the inner openness of the "heart" and their ultimate merging and identity remains a significant theme in Indian thought, especially in Saivism[14]. Surendranath Dasgupta further elucidates the 'inner' and 'outer' spatial relationship in Saiva philosophical traditions: in the philosophy of Abhinavagupta, which incorporates the Saivite traditions of Kashmir, the term *prakāsā* stands for the primeval and transcendent ubiquity of the "space" of consciousness. In Srikantha's

Saivite commentary on the *Brahmasūtra*, we hear about *cidākāsa*, the *ākāsa* of awareness, the power and potential of consciousness (*cicchakti*) which underlies and pervades the entire universe.[15] The element of air does not have an independent status of existence in Indian philosophical systems: air, by its origin, is correlated to space and time. Despite the difference between the schools and approaches, the interconnection between *vayu,* air, and *akasa,* space, is one of the most important underlying concepts in almost all the aesthetic and philosophical traditions in India. *Ayam ākāsa* is the extended world outside and *Antarhrdaya ākāsa* is the inner space of consciousness; the air element in the form of breath in the body connects these two spaces. The basic epistemological assumptions of *Sāmkhya*, *Yoga* and other systems of thought presented in the Saiva tradition, are firmly based on the correlation between breath and the 'inner space' of consciousness. Similarly, Abhinavagupta's interpretation of *rasa* clarifies the existence of 'inner' and 'outer' spaces in terms of the experience of *rasa* as an extension of Srikantha's Saivite concept of *cidākāsa*, the inner space of self awareness. Breath as the temporal element of the body connecting the inner and outer levels of consciousness is the key underlying idea presented in the Saivite philosophy. A further investigation, therefore, is required to establish the links between breath and consciousness, which will be the major focus of Chapter four.

2.3.1 Space and Time in *Sāmkhya*

Time, as presented in *Sāmkhya* epistemology, is a series of successive moments. A moment, for instance, is the smallest limit of duration, called *ksana*, which is the time taken by an atom in its motion of leaving its former position in space to reaching another point. This uninterrupted flow of moments constitutes the order of successive 'appearances' in space and time. Pulinbihari Chakravarti further explains this *Sāmkhya* view: our understanding of the world or the 'real' is based upon this 'smallest unit of infinite duration' of moments.[16] Previous and succeeding moments have no independent existence. Rather, what follows is the continuation of the previous moment. Hence, what exists in the present is only the present moment because two moments cannot co-exist. Present time, in this sense, is a time-sequence in which the previous moment is included. According to Chakravarti, this "is one of the fundamental doctrines of *Sāmkhya* that a manifest entity undergoes changes in every succeeding moment."[17] Past and future are considered as two variations of the ever-changing entity of the present moment. This spatio-temporal relationship is the basic underlying principle activating the cosmic structure, and, according to *Yoga Bhashya* (III. 53), the Yogins of superior power perceive the same cosmic motion within their body. *Yukti-dipika,* another classical text of *Sāmkhya*, further clarifies the link between the cosmos and the body in terms of time. As the universe owes its origin to time and flows continuously as an active process, the same cosmic rhythm can be found within the body, in the beating of the pulse and the solar and lunar circles of breathing.[18] *Yoga* classifies human respiration into two categories of sun and moon, and the analogy of the cosmic body is elaborately discussed in various classical texts which I will refer to in the following sections. The beating of the pulse is the most primordial movement of the body before the first inhalation of breath and hence, from the viewpoints of *Sāmkhya* and *Yoga*, pulsation and the flow of breath are the substratum of the human body which indicate the passage of time. In Sanskrit, *Kāla* refers to time. *Ahirbudhnya Samhitā* (51.42), a further ancient text of *Sāmkhya*, regarded *kāla*, time, as one of the aspects of *śakti*, energy; Devala, in the *Mahābhāsya* (xii. 275. 5), in his brief exposition of the eminence of time, acknowledged the previous view by extending the idea that time plays an important role in the emergence of the cosmos.[19] *Sāmkhya* and *Yoga* thus regarded energy and time as the most important aspects of supreme power located in the body.

Time and energy are, therefore, the causes of integration and disintegration of the entire cosmic structure, and are inseparable from each other. *Yoga*, in practice, subsumes this philosophical idea of the integration of time and energy as the 'union' of *prakrti* (nature) and *purusa* (self) mediated by breath. All the breath-related practices found in different traditions of *Yoga* are in effect techniques of exploring the potential energy level of the body by manipulating the temporal dimensions through various nostril operations. The idea of space is presented as a relative mechanism in *Sāmkhya* and *Yoga* because space is conceived in relation to time. *Sāmkhya-Sutra* (II. 12) makes it clear that both time and space are the products of ether.[20]

Sāmkhya and *Yoga* further provide examples of how epistemological understanding of the links between time, space and consciousness is practiced in the spiritual tradition of *Yoga* by combining the psycho-physical levels of the body. The following section will demonstrate how the physicality of breath is understood in *Sāmkhya*.

2.3.2 Breath and *Sāmkhya*

The integration of time and space is discussed extensively in *Sāmkhya* and *Yoga* in relation to breath, vitality and the cosmology of the body. The characteristic features of human embodiment lie in its capacity to perform the internal and external vital operations of the body, including its neurological functions. According to *Sāmkhya,* the body's vital operations are performed by five forms of breath called: *prana, apana, samana, udana and vyana.* These forms of breath are different modifications of the element of air, which incites the entire functioning of the system by bringing all the internal and external organs into action. This view is expressed by Vācaspati, in his *Tattva-vaiśāradī* (Y.S. III) and substantiated by Sankara, the renowned exponent of the Vedanta school, in his commentary on *Brahma-sūtra* (Y. S. 34).[21] These five vital forms of breath and their functions in the body are elaborately discussed in various texts of *Sāmkhya* and *Yoga* as follows:

1. *Prana* is located in the chest and extends up to the mouth and the nose through which air is drawn in and then expelled from the lungs. This breath is associated with the respiratory system and the living human body is the physical manifestation of *prana.*

2. *Apana's* sphere is down from the navel to the soles of the feet. It is associated with the excretory system of the body and concerned with the removal of waste. It also carries the foetus downward and, to a certain extent, helps the delivery of the child. This breath is said to be stronger than *prana* because it drags *prana* downward with the intention of limiting its scope.

3. *Samana* is situated between *prana* and *apana* and its sphere of activity extends down from the chest to the navel. Samana is

`tronger than the other two forms of breath because it attempts to keep a proper balance between the pressures of the drawing in of *prana* and the drawing out of *apana*. The psychological function of this form of breath is the feeling of pleasure, pain and other emotions. This breath is predominantly activated when a person is involved in group activities and performance.

4. *Udana* is located in the fore-part of the nose and extends its sphere up to the head. *Udana* carries chyle and other fat droplets upward. It is also connected with the arterial pulsations of the body. *Udana* is regarded as the most important form of breath in *yogic* terms because it drags the spirit from the lower level to the upper level. The natural flow of this form of breath is always obstructed by the activities of speech, verse and other compositions, through the opening of the mouth. The natural tendency of *Udana* is always to subdue other forms of breath by dragging them upward. Any feeling of superiority that a person may have is due to the external manifestation of this breath. The superiority of *Udana* to other forms of breath can be illustrated by the posture which a man takes up whenever he draws the sword from its sheath. This form of breath will be most active in the practice of martial arts.

5. *Vyana* is diffused throughout the system by circulating blood and other fluids evenly all over the body. This form of breath is also associated with the nervous system. Any acute feeling of inseparable connection or strong union between individuals arises as the result of the external manifestation of this form of breath. As long as this form of breath penetrates and functions properly within the system, all other forms of breath work in perfect harmony with the body. But whenever *Vyana* ceases to function properly, the result will be the gradual collapse of the entire system.

In *Sāmkhya* literature, the functions of these five forms of breath together with the sensory organs, the motor organs and the psychological conditions of the mind are conceptualised together as *prānāstak*, the eight constituents of vitality. Since a particular form of breath is related to specific organs of the body, there are systems described in *Yoga*, *Ayurveda*, the medical practice developed in the Sanskrit tradition, and the *Marmasutra*, the medical practice based on vital points in the body called *marmas* developed in Tamil tradition, of South India to explain the indications of the collapse of the system and death by examining the condition of breath and its physical effects on the body. The Indian system of reading pulsation, called *Nadisastra,* prescribed in *Ayurveda*, offers a more subtle understanding of the functioning of breath in the body, outlining all the merits and demerits of the system. More information can be found in the *Marmasutra* of South India but, unfortunately, due to its restricted practice and the unfamiliarity of the language in which the manuals are composed, a large domain of knowledge is either not understood properly or has disappeared from today's practice. The classifications of different physiological forms of breath in this section show the existence of a systematic knowledge produced by *Sāmkhya*. In the following section, I will look at how *Upanishads* have incorporated breath-related knowledge and practice.

2.3.3 Breath and the *Upanishads*

Vedas (1500 BC) and *Upanishads* (800-400 BC) are the sacred texts composed in Sanskrit, which are regarded as the voluminous containers of theological and philosophical literature and various other forms of knowledge and practices across the disciplines, ranging from human physiology to astronomy, from the art of warfare to highly sophisticated philosophical thinking. The *Vedas*, which are four in number—*Rik*, *Sama*, *Yajur* and *Atharva*—are mainly composed of hymns, instructions regarding rites, ceremonies and rules about the ways in which they should be conducted. The *Upanishads* are concerned with the highest aspects of several systems of knowledge. The word *Upanishad* literally means "sitting near", which conveys the idea of learning lessons in close proximity to the teacher. The word also means "secret teaching" because the purpose of an *Upanishad* is to disclose and explain the highly complex nature of ideas presented in various philosophical traditions, including *Vedas*. In this sense, *Upanishads* demonstrate the essence of Indian philosophical teachings and practices. As Sankara, the seventh century commentator of the

Vedanta school suggests, *Upanishads* hold the knowledge of Brahman—the knowledge that destroys the bonds of ignorance and leads to the highest goal of freedom.[22] This is 'knowledge' in a different sense that it is the unmediated and direct awareness, which engages with the unmanifested potentiality rather than linguistic and historical levels of meaning. How many *Upanishads* were written is unknown but one hundred and eight have been preserved. Of the one hundred and eight *Upanishads*, sixteen were recognised by Sankara as authentic and he wrote elaborate commentaries on ten of these from the perspective of Advaita Vedanta. *Upanishads* are also called Vedanta, which literally means the "end of *Vedas*". The name suggests the idea that the growth of the philosophical thinking presented in *Vedas* came to its zenith in the *Upanishads*. My intention in this section is to read selected relevant *Upanishads* in order to understand the ways in which breath is deciphered and debated in the terms of their philosophical and spiritual enquiry. This section will also demonstrate some breath-related practice described in the *Upanishads*, which will further contribute to my arguments, in the following sections, that the key focus of Indian spirituality is based on the psycho-physical implications of breath.

The cosmic vision presented in the *Upanishads* suggests the existence of *Brahman*, which is best understood, according to its various interpretations, as the unmanifest field of potential energy from which the existence of material forms emerged. The process of this emergence of the material universe of forms, names and sounds is the origin of the emergence of individual consciousness. Hence, the existence of the origin of an unmanifest level of consciousness is the most frequently articulated and debated epistemological question in Indian thought and surrounds the philosophical discourse of the *Upanishads*. The basic Upanishadic assumption is that the multitude of things and events are but different manifestations of the same ultimate 'reality' and this reality is called *Brahman*. This ultimate reality is understood as the inner essence of all things, which is infinite and beyond all concepts. It can neither be comprehended by the intellect nor can it be described in words. It is "beginningless, supreme: beyond what is and beyond what is not" (*Bhagavad Gita*: 4: 42). According to the *Chandogya Upanishad*, all creations emerge from *Brahman*; *atman*, the individual self is also the manifestation of this ultimate reality: "that is reality. That is *atman.* That art thou." (6.9.4). Fritjof Capra, evaluating this Upanishadic view in terms of modern astrophysics, concludes, in his terms, that the Hindu cosmic vision is based on the assumption that the existence of the entire universe depends on the play *(Lila)* of dynamic forces.[23] Capra argues further that the physical manifestation of the world is an illusion (*maya)* because it is ever-changing, based on the ultimate reality of *Brahman*: everything changes except *Brahman.* This entire motion of never-ending transformation involved in the existence of the universe is called *Karma*. *Karma* means action and "it is the active principle of the play in which everything is dynamically connected with everything else: the total universe in action."[24] The *Bhagavad Gita* explains *Karma* as 'the force of creation' from which everything has life. The dynamic link between time and action is further explained in the *Bhagavad Gita*:

> All actions take place in time by the interrelating of the forces of nature, but the man lost in selfish delusion thinks that he himself is the actor (8.3)

These fundamental views of Indian philosophy are, according to Capra, highly intellectual and philosophical and without any mythical content. This intellectual and philosophical element of *time* in terms of the 'force of creation' has been brought down, by Indian spiritual tradition, from its cosmic level to the level of human psychology. Understanding how each object in this universe is connected to others in this ultimate flow of ever-changing time is considered as the finest form of knowledge which the individual can achieve, according to Indian religious philosophies.

Ralph Yarrow, in the context of theatre studies, explains the term *Brahman* as "the unmoving source of movement, the potential which gives rise to all forms and forming,"[25] which is the deepest level of reality. As he goes on, "*Brahman* is accessible as awareness, by merging the individual consciousness with it"[26] and the world is the play of forms. Quoting from Fritjof Capra, Yarrow further argues that both modern quantum physicists and Eastern mystics view the material world as a vibrating movement of rhythmic patterns, which is defined by nuclear structures: the universe is not static but a constant dynamic stability between opposing forces. Similarly, Daniel Meyer

Dinkgräfe, in the context of a study of consciousness in the approaches of Indian acting, proposes *Brahman* as "a field of the absolute …the source of all possible qualities of manifestation,"[27] which is infinite and beyond space and time. However, this absolute is dynamic and includes opposing movements of qualities within itself, which interact with each other. The interaction of these opposing qualities is "responsible for the expression of *Brahman* into all aspects of creation as we experience, observe, know and discover it…all aspects of theatre, too, have their origin in this field of *Brahman*."[28] Yarrow's and Meyer-Dinkgräfe's views are supported by contemporary consciousness studies, as well as by the Advaita Vedanta philosophy of Sankara as commented on by Maharishi Mahesh Yogi.

What is *Brahman* and what is its nature? What are the ways in which one can experience it? These are the questions often asked in the *Upanishads*. In several *Upanishads*, questions about the existence of *Brahman* are asked directly in the form of a request, enquiring whether there is an existing system or a method or a practice which can be used in order to understand and experience it properly. The references in the *Upanishads* to a particular method seem to be directed towards some practice related to breath. Hence, breath and *Brahman* are interconnected in the *Upanishads*: the level of pre-expressive *Brahman* can be experienced through specific breath-related practices. The *Mandukya Upanishad* explains the nature of *Brahman* as the all pervading source, which is invisible, immortal and subtle, and which gives birth to the universe (I: 6). Forms emerge from *Brahman*, from its ever-expanding movement, and forms also submerge within it in the due course of the same movement, like a spider spreading out and folding up its web from its belly (I: 7&8). The physical manifestation of *Brahman* is thus illustrated in the *Mandukya Upanishad* as the entire universe including earth, animals, birds, plants, human beings and *prana* and *apana,* the two forms of breath, emerge from it (II. 7-10). This *Brahman* is the underlying dynamic force of the universe, which moves in the micro-structure of *anu,* the atom. The explanations of *Brahman* in the *Mandukya Upanishad* further clarify that this is the same principle that moves as the dynamics of the body. As the *Mandukya Upanishad* puts it, *Brahman* stays in the body (III. 7). The existence of *Brahman* in the body is experienced through a specific practice of meditation. One might ask further questions related to the explanation of *Brahman,* such as: if it stays in the body, exactly where does it stay? What is its nature and through which practices can one realise *Brahman?* As the questions are addressed in the further sections of the *Mandukya Upanishad*, the most underlying dynamic force of the body cannot be understood through words or sight. The animation of the body and the emergence of the mind are the physical manifestations of *Brahman* which uses five vital forms of breath as its tools (III. 9). Perception and emotions are functions of the mind and the result of the bodily operations of the five vital forms of breath provides the knowledge of the potential energy level in the body. Hence, breath is the most effective tool, according to the *Mandukya Upanishad*, for controlling the activities of the mind (perception and emotion) in order to understand the unmanifest level of potential energy in the body (III. 9-10). As the *Mandukya Upanishad* suggests, the source of potential energy in the body is associated with a gland, which is located in a specific zone. The location is described in the *Mandukya Upanishad* as the point inside the head where all the nerves in the body terminate, or the point inside the head from which the whole psycho-physical system is controlled (II. 6). This place is the seat of *Brahman* and, according to various Upanishadic sources, the only way to understand the level of *Brahman* is to do meditation through the sounds of AUM.

Let us look at this idea more closely as it is presented in the *Mandukya Upanishad*, in order to bring more clarity to it. Firstly, the *Mandukya Upanishad* says that *Brahman* is the unmanifest potential energy from which the universe emerges through a bi-polar movement. The second assumption is that this is the same source which is manifest in the body as perception and emotions, using five vital forms of breath as its tool. Thirdly, the *Mandukya Upanishad* says that *Brahman* is located in the inside of the head at a junction where all the nerves meet together, and, through the practice of meditating with AUM, one can reach the level of *Brahman*. All these ideas are recurrent themes discussed in several *Upanishads* and in various other texts of *Yoga* and *Marma* therapy. The location of *Brahman* in the body, the junction of nerves inside the head and the practice of AUM, all need to be looked at in more detail in order to identify a system based on breath.

The letters A-U-M are the symbolic representation of the primordial power which is operating constantly in the cosmic structure. This primordial cosmic power is the potential energy created by the two cosmic principles of *Nada* and *Bindu.* Sir John Woodroffe explains, in the *Garland of Letters*, that *Nada* and *Bindu* are the material cause of the universe established in the form of movement and stillness.[29] *Nada* literally means the seminal sound, which functions as the basis of all forms of words, which is the first going forth of a massive force of movement. *Bindu* literally means a dot or a point, which is the unmanifest potential energy—the infinitude—from which the force of *Nada* emerges out of a subtle micro-cosmic explosion. Hence, the universe is created from *Bindu,* the unmanifest energy, through the movement of *Nada,* the seminal sound, as the result of a micro-cosmic explosion. The letters A-U-M thus represent the cosmic principles of movement, form and energy illustrated as creative building, destructive disintegration and the holding of these two opposing forces in equilibrium. According to Woodroffe, the ideas presented in modern Western science as anabolism and catabolism in biochemistry, and as 'matter' as a relatively stable form of energy in physics, both explicate the same principles.[30] In the *Dhyanabindu Upanishad,* we see this cosmic principle of A-U-M further explained in terms of the body by saying that the body is a well-ordered cosmos manifested through the dynamic operation of *Bindu* and *Nada* (I: 1-9) in which *Brahman* is settled. In this *Upanishad* A-U-M are not only the three characteristic sounds of the primordial energy principle but also the three distinctive nostril operations through which the source energy of the physical manifestation is understood.

As the *Dhyanabindu Upanishad* further explains this in the context of *pranayama,* the drawing in of the air through the left nostril, called *puraka,* is the creative building and the exhalation of the air through the right nostril, called *recaka,* is the destructive disintegration; whereas, *kumbhaka,* the holding of the air in between these two bi-polar movements, holds the equilibrium of the body (I: 18-21). Several methods of *pranayama* are described in this *Upanishad* as means through which the fundamental energy principle of the cosmo-body is exposed. The *Brahmavidya Upanishad* suggests that the bodily locations of each syllable of A-U-M are successively

'A', situated two inches below the navel, 'U', in the middle of the chest and 'M', located further up in the mouth behind the uvula. Hence, the practice of A-U-M suggests a particular breath-related practice. The *Nada* is the flow of air and the *Bindu* is the unmanifest energy in the body. Individual consciousness emerges due to the bi-polar movements of breath taking place in the body and there is no sense of consciousness before the movement of breath, the *Nada,* takes place in the body. *Bindu* is explained in the *Mandukya Upanishad* as *Brahman*, the unmanifest potential energy from which the universe emerges through a bi-polar movement. The most important information we gain from the *Mandukya Upanishad* in the context of our discussion is that breath causes the emergence of individual consciousness.

In the *Taittiriya Upanishad*, we see a clear picture of the bodily location of the potential energy source (*Brahman* or *Purusha*): it is described as located inside the mouth at the back, and even inside and further up from the soft palate called uvula (VI: 1-2). As the *Upanishad* further explains, there is a place called *Brahmarantra*, where a *Nadi* called *Sushumna,* comes from the bottom of the spine to join with other important nerves. When a person takes her/his last breath, unlike in normal breathing, the breath is pulled upward and terminates finally inside the *Brahmarantra* and diffuses there with great joy (VI: 2). One who does not know about the path leading up towards *Brahmarantra,* and one who does not know the ways in which breathing can be directed towards *Brahmarantra*, might struggle to reach the place of endless joy (VI: 2). Thus the Taittiriya *Upanishad* suggests that we should learn the practice in order to understand, experience and make use of the unmanifest potential energy in the body located in the *Brahmarantra.* In the *Sangitaratnakara*, a text by Sarangadeva, the *Brahmarantra* is explained as the cerebral aperture, which is crucial to breath-related techniques in terms of exploring the dormant vital energy of the body (I: II: 153c-155b). Agastiya's *Marmasastra* further explains and clarifies the bodily location, nature and functioning of the potential energy source of the body in more physiological terms, which will be discussed in the following sections. There are several sections in the Taittiriya *Upanishad* which clearly uphold the connection between breath and the vital energy source of the body by saying that breath is the most important tool of practice to explore the potential energy concealed within the body (B.V: VI.1).

Looking at some of the breath-related instructions presented in the *Upanishads*, the *Swetasvatara Upanishad* illustrates a breath-related practice as:

> An intelligent man shall practice while keeping the body erect and then bringing the head, chest and throat parallel to it. There shall not be any thoughts or emotions; there shall only be a pure force of vital energy circulating in the body, which would enable you to control thousands of horses drawing a chariot; and there shall be an undisturbed mind in harmony with the body. When you feel like coming back, respire through your nostrils. (II. 8-9).

Similarly, in the *Brahmavidya Upanishad*, we see another clear demonstration of the practice as:

> The position of *Brahma* is located in the body at a distance of 12 *angula* from the tip of the nose. This is the place where the Yogins always belong. That is the place where the flow of breath defuses and disappears. Once you know how to bring your breath there, you can bring your mind there; once you bring your mind there, there is only joy without a comparison: you do not see even if you look at things and you do not feel anything even if your mind moves on to things. This is a secret. (I: 45).

This *Upanishad* lists ten forms of breath by adding five more vital forms of breath to the existing five proposed in *Sāmkhya*: they are *nagam, kurmam, krikaram, devadettam* and *dhananjayam*. The functions and bodily locations of these forms of breath are not mentioned anywhere in the *Upanishads* to which I refer in this chapter. Such further explanations related to the latter five forms of breath can be found, however, in the seminal texts of South Indian Siddha philosophy, like the *Thirumantiram* and the *Marmasastra*. I will discuss about these texts in details in the following sections. The *Brahmavidya Upanishad* also mentions *Vajrakumbhaka Sadhana* as one of the most important breath practices through which the practitioner can enter into the area of *Brahmarantra,* said to be the secret place of the highest form of joy and the source of potential energy.

Accounts of breath-related practices are widely available in several *Upanishads* like *Aitareya, Swetasvatara, Brahmavidya, Subala, Kshurika, Nadabindu,* the *Dhyanabindu* and *Yogatatva* and rather than demonstrating all the descriptions in detail, the scope of this section is limited to bringing together key ideas of breath-related practice described in them. In all these *Upanishads*, there is a similarity in the usage of words when the practice is described: *penetration of breath, upward direction, diffusing of breath, disappearance of breath, stillness, submergence into.* All these terms are movement-related words and suggest the existence of a clearly defined practice.

As we see in this section, the fundamental enquiry in Indian philosophy and spiritual practice, as it is presented in the *Upanishads*, justifies the implications of breath being at the centre of its thinking and practice. Breath is the bi-polar movement of temporality identical to cosmic motion in which the physical universe emerges from the potential field of unmanifest energy called *Brahman*. Breath is the creator of individual consciousness. This basic assumption, proposed by various *yogic* traditions suggests that the levels of individual consciousness can be controlled through the manipulation of breath. All breath-related practices use *time* as a basic tool in altering the levels of consciousness as well as to explore the vital energy of the body. *Upanishads* contain specific breath-related practices but it is very difficult to understand these systems because they are not in practice nowadays. The South Indian Siddha tradition is thus important in this context to help decipher the Upanishadic knowledge related to the philosophy and practice of breath. The *Upanishads* establish links between micro-cosmic and macro-cosmic by describing air as the movement of the 'force of creation', connecting elements of the emergence of cosmic world. Similarly, the *Upanishads* link the body and consciousness by using breath as a temporal force through which *Brahman*, the timeless infinitude, is experienced. The *Upanishads* thus offer descriptions of various breath-related practices as means of realizing the level of consciousness beyond time (*Brahman*). However, those descriptions of practice hardly explain the system and therefore, I desire to extend my investigations into other physical approaches like *Yoga* and

Ayurveda aiming to identify some practice related to the descriptions that I gathered theoretically.

2.4 Breath in *Yoga* and *Ayurveda*

The word *Yoga* is derived from the Sanskrit root *yuj*, which means 'to direct', but the meaning commonly understood is union or communion. The Latin *jungere, jugum* and the French *joug* also have the same meaning. *Yoga* is the fourth of the six systems of Indian philosophy—the others are *Nyaya*, *Vaisheshika*, *Sāmkhya*, *Karma Mimansa* and *Vedanta*. Further to this classification, the core of Indian philosophy is based on "four interdependent concepts of 'kinetic ideas' such as *karma, māya, Brahman* and *Yoga*."[31] The law of *karma* is the law of universal causality, which connects man with the cosmos and condemns him to transmigrate indefinitely. The dynamic process that creates and maintains the cosmos is the principle of illusion, which is *māya* because stability is an illusion of ignorance (*avidyā*) within the eternal motion and growth of the universe: things are in the flux of an ever-changing state. The concept of *Brahman* is absolute reality which is unmanifest and out of which the cosmic illusion and *karma*, causality, emerge. This state of *Brahman* is unconditioned and indestructible. Finally, *Yoga* is the means to understand the interdependency of all other 'kinetic ideas.' Generally speaking, the word *Yoga* serves to designate certain techniques and methods of practice relating to body, mind and breath, which ultimately lead to a state of liberation from universal causalities and cosmic illusion, through understanding the all pervading 'kinetic principle' located in the body. According to Eliade, Patanjali's *Yoga* Sutras are:

> The result of an enormous effort not only to bring together and classify a series of ascetic practices and contemplative formulas ...but also to validate them from a theoretical point of view by establishing their bases, justifying them, and incorporating them into a philosophy.[32]

The main object of *Yoga* practice is *ekāgratā*, which is explained by Patanjali as a process of psycho-physical attention towards an object or an idea or a thought or the infinity obtained by integrating the psycho-physical faculties.[33] The practice of concentration tends to control two mental activities: the sense activity (*indriya)* and the activity of the sub-conscious (*samskāra*). Control means the ability to intervene at will and directly in order to enhance the bio-mental activities. This kind of concentration can be achieved through numerous exercises and techniques in which physicality plays a crucial role. One cannot, for instance, obtain concentration if the body is in an uncomfortable posture or if the respiration is disorganised or unrhythmic. Hence, according to Patanjali, *yogic* techniques involve several classifications such as: 1. restraints (*yama),* 2. disciplines (*niyama*), 3. bodily attitudes and postures (*asanas),* 4. rhythmic respiration (*pranayama*), 5. emancipation of sensory activity from the domain of exterior objects (*pratyahara*), 6. concentration (*dharana*), 7. *yogic* meditation (*dhyana),* 8. s*amadhi*. These are called the eight limbs of *Yoga* and each section of practice has specific psycho-physical purposes that are discussed at length in various classic texts. As Iyengar explains,[34] the first of these limbs is concerned with disciplines relating to the maintenance of ethical and social values and the second is concerned with the rules of conduct that apply to individual disciplines concerning health and cleanliness. The third limb of *Yoga*, the physical postures, brings mental and physical strength to the body. *Pranayama,* the fourth limb, is concerned with various methods in which breath is manipulated and controlled in the body in order to strengthen the nervous system and cultivate vital energy. The fifth stage of *Yoga* is to bring the mental activities under control by controlling the respiration of breath. *Dharana,* the sixth stage is obtaining a perfect state of concentration in psycho-physical activities and the seventh stage is concerned with meditation in which various physical and breath-related techniques are employed in order to explore the unknown capacities of body and mind. Finally, the state of *Samadhi* is said to create contact with the potential source energy located in the cosmology of the body.

All these eight limbs are the major focus of discussion in all the available systems of *Yoga* and aim to explain the nature of the psycho-physicality of human embodiment. To mention a few examples in relation to breath, according to Yogi Ramacharaka,[35] human respiration takes place in the four following ways: 1. high breathing, 2. mid breathing, 3. low breathing, and 4. complete breathing. High breathing, also referred to as clavicular breathing, uses only the upper part of the chest and lungs; in mid breathing, also referred to as rib breathing or intercostal breathing, the diaphragm is pushed upward and the abdomen drawn in. Low breathing, also known as abdominal or diaphragmatic breathing, achieves a healthy system in breathing by bringing the diaphragm into use. Diaphragmatic breathing is mentioned in all the *yogic* systems as an important approach to respiration. This is also called 'bellows breathing.' As Dhirendra Brahmachari suggests, this system of breathing is deep and rapid with a sharp and quick intake and outlet of breath, which accompanies the kind of noise which a pair of bellows would make operated.[36] Iyengar extensively describes over 200 *Yoga* postures and fourteen different techniques of breathing exercises which he developed from various classical texts like the *Hatayoga-Pradipika,* the *Gheranda-Samhita* and the *Yogachudamani Upanishad.* The following sections are illustrations of the knowledge of breath available in *Yoga*, presented in two seminal texts, the *Sangitaratnakara* by Sarangadeva and the *Siva Svarodaya Shastra.* Both the texts were written in Sanskrit. The *Sangitaratnakara* is the classical text on music written by Sarangadeva. While explaining the genesis of human embodiment as the instrument of music, Sarangadeva offers a coherent illustration of the links between the body and breath. The *Siva Svarodaya Shastra* is another classical text on *Yoga*, whose author is unknown, and the original text is hardly available (I have seen neither the original text nor the translation of it. Rather, I use a text written on the basis of the original Sanskrit text). I choose these two texts because of the quality and the coherence of information they provide. Furthermore, the *Sangitaratnakara* comprises *Ayurveda*'s medical assumptions about the human body and breath whereas the *Siva Svarodaya Shastra* consists of *tantric* and *yogic* practices related to breath: all these strands are practice-based and therefore, highly useful to the investigations of this thesis.

2.4.1 The *Sangitaratnakara* and the Genesis of the Human Embodiment

The *Sangitaratnakara* is a monumental work on the science of musical art composed by Sarangadeva, the king of Kashmir and a renowned scholar in Sanskrit, whose period is dated back to 12 A.D. The elaborate description of the human embodiment, derived from *Ayurveda* and *Yoga*, presented in this text in the context of music, is one of the most fascinating elements of the *Sangitaratnakara*. According to the synoptical view of Sarangadeva, *Nada,* the primary cause of the phenomenal world, is the basis of the art of music. The *Nada* is twofold: the produced (*Ahata)* and the unproduced (*Anahata*). The former is an object of sense perception whereas the latter is a matter of the experience of *Yoga*. Sarangadeva considered music as the perceptual manifestation of *Nada* produced by the body (II: A: ii). The human body is the mediator in this process of making the unmanifest *Nada* into the perceptual form of music. Sarangadeva's views on the physical body can be classified into three categories: metaphysical, physiological and psychophysical.

A. The Metaphysical Viewpoint

Sarangadeva's metaphysical view considers the human body as the physical manifestation of a universal substance and *Nada* as the very basis of all manifest life. As he further explains the link between *Nada* and the phenomenal world, "*Nada* manifests letters (of alphabets); letters constitute words, and words make a sentence; so, the entire business of life is carried on through language" (II: A: i). *Jiva,* the individual being is the derivation of *Brahman,* the timeless 'cosmic reality', through the process of creation. The process of creation is based on *maya,* illusion, because all physical manifestations are subject to specific modes of perceptual time and space. The perception of a specific mode of time and space is relative in the wider context of universal space and time and therefore, physical manifestations naturally occupy a limited space and time. This specific perception of a limited sense of space and time is characteristic to individual perception and individual consciousness, in this sense, is limited to a perceptual mode of space and time. The illusion of creation is mediated through *karma,* action. Governed by the laws of action (*karma*), virtuous as well as evil, productive of pleasure and of pain, the individual self experiences life through a physical body. The phenomenon is essentially transitory, comes into being, continues for a certain time and returns to its source. This source, which is the substratum of the ephemeral world, is beyond time, and eternal. Hence, the phenomenon of the world is created out of the measurelessness of eternity and is dissolved back into it. This is the eternal *play* of the laws of *karma* (action), according to Sarangadeva, which continues eternally (II: B: iv).

According to the metaphysical basis of reality elucidated by Sarangadeva, the phenomenal world is created through five basic elements called *mahabhuta*: the first of these elements is *akasa*, which is the objective reality that is the substratum of sound perceived by the ear; *vayu* denotes the element through which the perception of touch takes place; *tejas* is the element that is responsible for the perception of colour; *jala* is the element that is responsible for the perception of taste; *prthivi*, finally, is the element that produces the perception of odour. The physical universe is created by these basic elements on the basis of five types of perception and the embodied self is, therefore, closely connected to this universal principle.

B. The Physiological Viewpoint

This viewpoint allows an elaborate account of human physiology and the major topics Sarangadeva discusses from this perspective include: the development of the embryo; the birth of the child; the physical development of the body, including the formation of memory and the development of intellect; the functions of breath in the body; the constitution and the organs of the body; skins and membranes; tissues and receptacles; states of consciousness; the nine canals and the bones; their number and types; muscles; the number of arteries and veins; the number of major and minor vessels of vital essence; the vital parts of the body; the number of hairs on the body; and the measure of fluids in the human body. Starting from describing the various stages through which the embryo develops during the entire period of pregnancy, Sarangadeva conducts a useful comparative study of the monumental works of Indian medicine and surgery written by Caraka and Susruta. Since most of these detailed descriptions of human physiology are irrelevant to my thesis, I intend to give only a brief account of the way in which Sarangadeva considers breath in the context of human physiology.

Sarangadeva discusses the role of breath in human embodiment in terms of the faculty of perception. Motion, for instance, is derived from air and there are five types of motion: upwards, downwards, contraction, linear movement and expansion. Sarangadeva also mentions ten modifications of air as breath and explains their different functions in the body. These ten forms of breath and their various functions in the body are commonly mentioned in several other texts of *Yoga*, the *Marmasastra* and the *Upanishads*. According to the theories of *Ayurveda*, sense perception takes place because of the fact that the senses as well as sense-objects are basically made out of the same material and hence there is a correlation between them. I would like to emphasise at this point that the *Sangitaratnakara* carefully establishes the connection between breath and motion. Both movement and breath are derived from air and both are temporal aspects that depend on each other. Each movement of the body contains a parallel movement of breath in the body and in reverse the movement of breath in the body animates the body. Both are interdependent elements functioning with crucial roles in the body. The formation of human consciousness and feelings are deeply interconnected to the temporality and movement of the body and mind. I highlight the connection of breath and motion established by Sarangadeva because the major discussion in the following chapters focus on temporality and nostril modes, which I have been developing from the beginning of this thesis. Sarangadeva further considers breath as a crucial element in explaining the physiological viewpoint of the body.

C. The Psychophysical Viewpoint

The *Sangitaratnakara*, while explaining the psychophysical view point of breath describes *Cakras*, the basic information derived from *Yoga*. Several schools of *Yoga* and Tantra propose six psychophysical centres in the body. These centres are said to be the centres of energy and consciousness and there are also systems of practice, suggested by *yogic* and *tantric* practices to cultivate enormous psychic and spiritual strength through manipulating those centres. The aim of *Yoga* is to train the mind to concentrate upon and penetrate all these six psychophysical centres to attain complete mastery over the psychophysicality of the human embodiment. This aim is individual liberation of consciousness from the limited senses of mind and matter. Whereas other texts describe six such *Cakras*, the *Sangitaratnakara* proposes ten. Those ten *Cakras* are: *Adhara Cakra,*

Svadhisthana Cakra, Manipuraka Cakra, Anahata Cakra, Visuddhi Cakra, Lalana Cakra, Ajna Cakra, Manas Cakra, Soma Cakra and *Sahasrapatra Cakra.*

The basic concept of *Cakra* suggests kinetic energy situated in the body, which can be aroused and properly cultivated throughout the body. This kinetic energy is said to be the vital energy, called *kundalini* in *yogic* terms. *Kundalini* is said to be asleep or in a static mood, in the form of a coiled snake, at the base *Cakra, Adhara Cakra,* which is also called *muladhara Cakra,* located in between the anus and the genitals. As Shringy and Sharma elucidate, when this slumbering energy is awakened, it rushes through the spinal cord to the next highest *Cakra* at very high speed, and the practitioner is expected to experience a different, heightened level of energy and consciousness.[37] According to various *tantric* and *yogic* systems, there are two ways in which the kinetic energy or *kundalini* can be aroused: through sounds and through breath. The approach employing sounds is called *Mantra-sadhana,* whereas the approach employing breath is called *Pranayama.* These approaches are based on two fundamental kinetic principles which are sound and movement, and the whole idea behind the concept of *kundalini* is that the energy can be produced within the body through sound and movements.

The word *Mantra* literally means 'calls forth', which also suggests the meaning of 'liberation through mental processes.'[38] *Man* of *Mantra* comes from the first syllable of *manana,* the Sanskrit word for thinking and *tra* comes from *trana* meaning liberation from the bondage of the phenomenal world. Hence, the word *Mantra* suggests the idea of a transition of consciousness from daily to extra-daily. A *Mantra* is composed of letters and these letters are arranged in a specific sequence of sounds of which the letters are the representative signs. Each *Mantra* is intoned in a particular way according to the letters and the rhythm and resonates in the body by vibrating in each zone of the body related to the respective letter of the alphabet. The *Mantra* in this way is the sound-body. In the theory accompanying a specific *tantric* practice called *Nyasa,* the physical human body is divided into 51 zones including *Cakras* that correspond to the 51 Sanskrit letters of vowels and consonants. The aim of *Mantra* is to stimulate the body's energy centres or *Cakras* by vibrating and combining one with another. For example, the significance of the syllable *aham,* if it forms part of a *Mantra*, is that it is composed of the letters *a* + *ha* with a connecting sound *m*, linking three major zones in the body. These zones are the *muladhara*, the base *Cakra*; *anahata,* the *Cakra* located on the chest; and *ajna,* the *Cakra* situated in the middle of the eyebrows. Hence, the word *aham* combines three bodily zones, and three *Cakras* through the resonance of the reinforcement and prolongation of sounds. Each *Mantra* consists of a pattern of breathing, though the reverberation of sound is more important in *Mantra* in terms of the energy levels of the body. *Ham* + *sa,* another *Mantra* suggests the breathing process consisting of inspiration and expiration: *sa* refers to inspiration and *ham* refers to expiration, but this expiration is rather known as internalisation (See Chapter four). Generating the sound energy by rendering letters and then transforming the energy into physical energy by reverberation at bodily zones is the underlying principle of *Mantra-sadhana* in terms of the vital energy of the body. *Mantra*s always affect the *Cakra*s. However, in the context of my research I have not been able to establish in detail the connection between *Cakras* and *Mantras*.

Pranayama is another approach of enlivening *Cakras.* Described in *Yoga*, the S*angitaratnakara* suggests a breath-related practice:

> Mounted upon the vital breath, the self conscious-entity through the *Sushumna* keeps on ascending to the cerebral aperture and descending back moving like a right rope dancer.[39]

The description of this breath-related practice shows Sarangadeva's familiarity with *Yoga*. The term *Sushumna,* technically refers to *Yoga*'s understanding of the existence of a middle path in human breathing. *Sushumna,* according to *Yoga* is the central most *Nadi* (tubular vessel) that proceeds from the end of the spinal column and opens into the cerebral aperture. The dormant creative energy, when awakened, rises up along this *Nadi.* The S*angitaratnakara* incorporates *ayurvedic*, *yogic* and *tantric* knowledge and practice in explaining the different functions of breath in the body. However, the S*angitaratnakara* does not provide any detailed description of the practices that are mentioned in the text though there are descriptions of breath-related practices borrowed from other disciplines. So, at this stage, it is highly important to the thesis to look at the *Siva Svarodaya*

Shastra, which explains the subtle and complex functioning of breath in the body. In this section, the *Sangitaratnakara* defines ten *Cakras* as the psycho-physical centres of the body and further says that *Cakras* can be enlivened through two processes: *Mantra sadhana* and *Pranayama*. The information provided in this section regarding *Cakras*, *Mantras* and the three predominant *Nadis* of breathing can be red as metaphors suggesting some complex psycho-physical dynamics within the body. *Cakras* are known as the physical locations of the body, where potential psycho-physical energy is situated. Several classical texts of *yoga,* music and *Ayurveda*, including *Upanishads* and *Sangitaratnakara*, suggest two practical approaches to explore the potential psycho-physical energy source within the body: vibrations of sounds through *mantras* and specific systems of breathing as subtle internal movements. According to these systems of knowledge, the forces and patterns of voiced sounds and breathing, like any other physical approach, vibrate and penetrate the physical energy centres of the body and generate a heightened psycho-physical energy level within the body. Similarly, *nadis* are explained in *Marmatherapy* as the tubular vessel, through which the *prana,* the life force, flows, and the physiological functions of *nadis* are further explained in the texts with incredible details (See the following section, 2.5.1, for further details). *Nadis* are similar to Chinese meridians, in this sense. However, the interconnections between the energy centres, sounds and breathing need to be verified on the pragmatic level of physiology as well as the psychological and consciousness levels of experience through further research. Since, this line of enquiry does not seem to have some direct and immediate impact into my thesis, in the following section I will look at the *yogic* tradition, presented in the *Siva Svarodaya Shastra* to figure out the practical base of breath aiming to understand the techniques by which the vital energy can be enlivened. The purpose of including some of the following sections like breath and astrology is only to show how breath has been incorporated into various systems of Shaivite practice though some of the claims seem to be highly unverifiable.

2.4.2. The *Siva Svarodaya Shastra* and the *Yogic* Techniques of Breathing

In the case of the *Siva Svarodaya Shastra*, both the author of the text and the period in which the text was composed are unknown. The text was originally written in Sanskrit and translations of the full text are available only in a couple of the regional languages in India. What is mostly available for English readers are books either written on a few aspects of the original texts or mentioning the existence of the original text in Sanskrit. My interviews with several people who are either researchers or practitioners of *Yoga* revealed that many of them have not seen the *Siva Svarodaya Shastra* but all of them have heard about the inaccessible existence of the text. In this section, I use two recent publications based on the *Siva Svarodaya Shastra* written by Harish Johari and Swami Sivapriyananda to illustrate the basic principles of this school of *Yoga*. The word *svara* literally means sound but in the context of breath it means the sound of breath. The word *udaya* means rise and hence *svara-udaya* means the rise of breath. As Sivapriyananda clarifies further, this is not a method of breath control but rather 'a way of using normal respiration to harmonise the forces of life with the pattern of breathing'[40] The technique of *svara-udaya* is based on the observable fact, which was frequently overlooked for centuries in *Yoga*, that we normally breathe freely through only one nostril at a time. The human respiratory system changes intermittently from one nostril to another, roughly every one and half hours and there is a qualitative difference between the breath in each persistent changeover. The breath that flows from the left nostril is cool, soothing, passive and feminine in nature, whereas the breath that flows from the right nostril is warm, energizing, active and masculine. According to the *svara-udaya* system, the left nostril is connected to the moon and the right nostril is connected to the sun; hence the change that takes place in nostril operations is said to be due to the movement of the solar and lunar cycles. The following sections provide information about the *svara-udaya* system of breathing.

A. Nostrils: Structure and Modes

The *svara-udaya* technique of breathing is known as the science of nasal breath, which deals with the relationship between the nasal breath and the subtle nerves of the body. The technique also operates within the understanding of respiration between lunar and solar cycles and the basic gross elements of the body.[41] As Johari explains the *svara-udaya* teachings further, the nose is the only organ which continuously interacts with external physical conditions. The rate of our breathing quickly responds to the changes in our physical and mental conditions. In anger, for example, breathing becomes fast, whereas in sleep it becomes slow and regular. An average human organism breathes one inhalation and one exhalation thirteen to fifteen times a minute, which means that an average human being breathes 21,000 to 21,600 times in a twenty-four-hour cycle. According to the *Siva Svarodaya Shastra,* the life span of a human organism is measured not in years but in number of forms of breath. At the rate of fifteen breaths per minute, a human life is comprised of a total of 946,080,000 breaths which is a full 120 years. To compare this with the number of breaths in other animals: a hare breathes 55 times per minute, an ape 30 times, a cat 24 times, a dog 15-18 times, a horse 8-12 times and a tortoise only 3 times a minute. The whole knowledge of breath and its various practices in the *Siva Svarodaya Shastra* is based on the assumption that since breath is deeply connected to the entire psychophysical system of the human organism, the methods of understanding through controlling and manipulating respiration will eventually create remarkable alterations in the levels of emotion and consciousness, including the psychophysical qualities of life.

Through a network of sensory nerves in the nose, the nostrils are connected to subtle nerves or *Nadis*. These *Nadi*s, according to Johari, are of two kinds:

1. Conduits of *pranic* force—*pranavaha Nadi.*
2. Conduits of psychic energy—*manovaha Nadi*

Some of the most important *Nadi*s carry both pranic energy, flowing as electromagnetic currents, and psychic energy, flowing as feeling, vibrations or frequencies, at the same time. There are fourteen important *Nadis*, the tubular vessels, that carry both kinds of energy and three out of fourteen are of vital importance according to Johari. These three *Nadis*, which are called *Ida, Pingala* and *Sushumna*, are connected to the limbic system. From a medical perspective, *Ida* influences the hypothalamus and the pituitary gland, activating the growth of hormones and the anabolic process. *Pingala* influences the thalamus and hypothalamus. The *Sushumna* is concerned with the corpus callosum and the cerebellum. When it bifurcates in the brain stem, one branch of the *Sushumna* goes to the corpus callosum, while the other, known as the posterior *sushumna*, passes through the cerebellum to the cerebral cortex and terminates in the corpus callosum. Here it joins with the other branch known as the anterior *sushumna*. This point of termination is called the fontanelle, the 'soft spot' in an infant's skull that hardens after three to six months. These three *Nadi*s, through their connection with the endocrine glands, influence the entire body chemistry and the chemical nature of the human organism. The *sushumna Nadi* is the only nerve that directly pierces all the *Cakras* or the physical centres of the subtle body. These centres are connected with the internal organs through sympathetic and parasympathetic nerves, which are connected to the autonomic nervous system working through the spinal column. The *sushumna* is thus connected with the network of sympathetic and parasympathetic nerves and the autonomic nervous system through its connection to the *Cakras* and its passage through the spinal column. Although the three *Nadis* meet at the same place in the pelvic plexus, they originate from different parts of the base of the spine. According to the *Siva Svarodaya Shastra*, all three of these *Nadis* can be activated and controlled through breath in order to control the chemical balance and the energy level of the body. The *Siva Svarodaya Shastra* explains the *Nadis* as follows:[42]

> *Ida*: This *Nadi* originates at the base of the spine and works as the left channel. It flows on the left side of the spinal column and terminates in the left nostril by branching into fine capillaries. This *Nadi* becomes active when breathing is carried out by the left nostril. In *yogic* terms, this nostril is known as feminine or maternal and it is connected with right hemisphere, making it emotional and magnetic in nature. Because of its dominance during the ascending cycle of the

moon, it is called lunar. The breath flowing through the left nostril is called *Ida* or moon breath.

Pingala: This *Nadi* originates at the base of the spine and acts as the right channel. It is situated on the right side of the spinal column and terminates in the right nostril by branching into fine capillaries. During the operation of the right nostril, this *Nadi* becomes active. It is connected with solar currents and its energy is considered to be masculine. The right nostril is connected with the left cerebral hemisphere, making it verbal and rational in nature. Because it is dominant during the descending cycle of the moon, it is called solar. The breath flowing through the right nostril is called *Pingala* or sun breath.

Sushumna: This *Nadi* originates at the base of the spine and is situated between the *Ida* and *Pingala*. It is also known as the central canal and its energy flows through the interior of the spinal column. It pierces the palate at the base of the skull and terminates at the top of the skull, at the soft spot. When air flows in both nostrils equally, the sushumna *Nadi* becomes active. It is fiery in nature. This *Nadi* usually works at dawn or dusk automatically, and also for short intervals when the transition from one nostril to the other nostril takes place. It is also said that all human beings breathe through both nostrils just before death, when *sushumna* becomes active.

These are the three modes of human respiration according to the *Siva Svarodaya Shastra* and the *pranayama,* the breathing techniques, in all *yogic* traditions are connected to different combinations of these three modes.

B. Nostrils and the Solar System

Each nostril mode is connected to lunar cycles and the *Siva Svarodaya Shastra* extensively documents the relationship. In the following discussion I follow Johari's descriptions in order to explain this complicated breath calendar.[43] The lunar cycle influences the fluids in the body and creates identifiable effects in the emotional levels of the body. Nostrils are directly connected to the cycles of the moon and during the ascending and descending cycles, the left and the right nostrils are alternatively dominant. In the ascending moon cycle, the left nostril operates for nine days, on lunar dates 1, 2, 3, 7, 8, 9, 13, 14 and 15. In the same cycle, the right nostril operates for six days, on lunar dates 4, 5, 6, 10, 11 and 12. In the descending moon cycle, the right nostril likewise operates for nine days, on lunar dates 1, 2, 3, 7, 8, 9, 13, 14 and 15. In the same cycle, the left nostril operates for six days, on lunar dates 4, 5, 6, 10, 11 and 12. The right nostril operates for nine days and the left for six days. To describe these operations more clearly:

1. The right nostril is associated with the solar planets: the Sun, Mars and Saturn. On the day corresponding to these planets - Sunday, Tuesday and Saturday - the right nostril works for one hour, starting ninety minutes before sunrise. Half an hour before sunrise it changes and the nostril of the day takes over. When the right nostril is also the nostril of the day, flow of breath through this nostril on these three days is auspicious.

2. The left nostril is associated with the lunar planets: the Moon, Mercury, Jupiter and Venus. On the days corresponding to these planets - Monday, Wednesday, Thursday and Friday - the left nostril works for one hour, starting ninety minutes before sunrise. Half an hour before sunrise the nostril of the day takes over. When the left nostril is also the nostril of the day, flow of breath through this nostril on these four days is auspicious.

3. The *Sushumna Nadi* is active when both nostrils function together. It automatically operates very briefly at dawn and dusk, when the nostril connected with the planet stops and the nostril of the day takes over. This *Nadi* is said not to be influenced by either the ascending or the descending cycles of the moon.

The same nostril that starts the day one hour before the sunrise also ends with the day at sunset. Day and night and the rise and setting of the Sun and Moon take place constantly in the human organism as a result of the constant interplay of left and right nostril modes. The entire chemical balance of the body is maintained through this constant interplay between nostril operations; the *Siva Svarodaya Shastra* claims that by changing nostril modes intentionally one can alter the level of consciousness and emotion by changing the chemical balance in the body. This needs to be researched properly in the contexts of both *yogic* knowledge and modern medicine in order to explore more connections between respiration and the body. To highlight a point for further discussion in the context of my argument in this thesis, these left and right nostril modes indicate the passage of time, whereas the middle path of *Sushumna* breathing does not suggest any time: it is timeless, or beyond the ordinary sense of time.

C. Techniques to Check Nostril Modes:

The Moon changes bi-monthly creating two cycles:

1. Ascending cycle, from new moon to full moon, when the moon is gradually increasing in size and influence.
2. Descending cycle, from full moon to new, when the moon is gradually decreasing in size and effect.

Hence, the *Siva Svarodaya Shastra* suggests specific methods by means of which the nostril operations can be checked bi-monthly. The following are the two ways of checking nostril operations suggested by the *Siva Svarodaya Shastra.*[44]

1. In the morning following the full moon, the descending moon cycle starts. The right nostril should operate for three consecutive days at dawn.

2. In the morning following the new moon, the ascending moon cycle starts at dawn and the left nostril should operate for three consecutive days.

The body maintains its natural, healthy rhythm if the nostrils are working properly. If the correct nostril is not working, there will be a change in the body chemistry and this alteration can lead to both physiological and psychological problems within the next two weeks.

According to the *Svara-udaya* system, it is therefore important to check and correct the problem at the outset and there are techniques available to activate the correct mode intentionally at any moment of time. The following are considered the correct modes of operation while checking the breath:

1. Right following the night of the full moon
2. Left following the night of the new moon

The nostril should be checked around dawn before getting out the bed and in the case of incorrect nostril dominance, the person should not get out of bed until it is brought back to its correct mode relating to the lunar cycle. It is also suggested that one should wait approximately ten to thirty minutes after the sun rises to change the nostril operation intentionally.

D. Techniques to Change Nostril Modes

The methods of changing the nostril modes are discussed in detail in the *Siva Svarodaya Shastra,* along with the ways of identifying the dominant nostril mode and suggestions regarding under what circumstances the nostril modes can be changed. The following are the three ways to identify the dominating nostril:

1. The dominant nostril will have an undisturbed flow of breath. Press one nostril and check which nostril is congested.

2. Breathe out quickly several times in a row without plugging both nostrils and you can feel a cool sensation in the dominant nostril.

3. Breathe out on a piece of glass or a mirror. The residual vapour will deposit on the side of the operating nostril.

When the middle path is dominant, you will feel either that both of your nostrils are free or that both are congested. The flow of breath will be even through both nostrils when the middle path dominates. The *Siva Svarodaya Shastra* suggests the three following methods to change the dominating nostrils whenever it is necessary (Johari: 1989, p.18):

1. Press the operating nostril gently with the thumb and breathe forcefully through the congested nostril.

2. Lie down on the side of the operating nostril. That is to say, lie down on the right side when the right nostril is operating and vice versa. Place a small cushion under the armpit bearing the weight to stimulate the nerve on that side. The nostril flow will change to the other side within a few minutes. And also note that when the person is healthy the nostril changes quickly but in case of chemical imbalance in the body it will take longer to change the nostril mode. If the person is ill, it will take an hour and more to change the operating nostril.

3. Sit in a comfortable posture and turn the gaze towards the congested nostril. This practice will be effective if combined with the first method.

Swami Sivapriyananda describes an ancient method which yogis traditionally use to change the operating nostril.[45] This method involves the use of the 'Y' shaped crutch-like instrument called the *Yoga-dandu.* Place this instrument under the armpit of the operating nostril and lean over and press it between the chest and the arm. The flow of the breath will change to the other side of the nostril within about 10 to 15 minutes with this course of action. This method is used by Yogins. Swami Sivapriyananda mentions the existence of a fifth, method; however, he does not describe it because one can learn this most delicate method only from a Guru who knows it and is willing to share it. I would say that what is known to the world at the moment in this context is very little and very general information about breath, compared to what is hidden amongst people who come from the *yogic* lineage.

Johari offers a brief description of when and under what circumstances the operating modes can be changed, according to the *Siva Svarodaya Shastra*:

1. If one feels disturbed, shows signs of illness, experiences an unusual taste in the mouth or a lack of energy.

2. If the right or left nostril operates for more than two or three hours in succession.

3. If the Moon nostril operates at the time the Sun nostril should normally be operating or vice versa.

4. If you want to do any activity related to the left and right nostrils when the middle path operates. Meditation and relaxation are the activities suggested when the middle path is in operation. (See the tables below)

Table 1. Qualities associated with the nostrils

Left Nostril	Right Nostril
Days: Monday, Wednesday, Thursday and Friday *Cycle*: Ascending Moon cycle *Influential levels:* * Ahead, left and above *Nature:* Magnetic, feminine, lunar, alkaline *Suitable for*: Peaceful activities, *Duration:* One to two hours *Connected with:* Right hemisphere of the brain; left side of the body. *Dominant:* Morning, following new moon night. *Sanskrit name:* Ida *Body Chemistry:* Mucus dominated	*Days*: Sunday, Thursday and Saturday. *Cycle*: Descending Moon cycle. *Influential levels:* * Behind, right and below *Nature:* Electrical, masculine, Solar, acidic. *Suitable for:* Difficult activities *Duration:* One to two hours. *Connected with:* Left hemisphere of the brain; right side of the body. *Dominant:* Morning following full moon night. *Sanskrit name:*Pingala *Body Chemistry:* Bile dominated

* Anyone positioned in these directions in relation to your body becomes subject to the influence of this nostril. In such a situation, gaining favours from the person or influencing his or her thoughts becomes easy (Johari: 1989, p. 26).

Table 2. Activities associated with the nostrils*

Left Nostril	Right Nostril
1. Stable business, requiring no movement.	1. Unstable business, requiring movement.
2. Long term activities	2. Temporary activities or jobs that can be accomplished quickly.
3. Journey to a far-off place.	3. Journey to a near place
4. Collection of ornaments	4. Return journey
5. Collecting food grains and necessities of life	5. Studying or teaching martial arts.
6. Beginning of study (Regular school education)	6. Studying hard skills and destructive sciences
7. Playing musical instrument	7. Writing manuscripts
8. Singing	8. Practice of Shastras
9. Learning to dance	9. Practice of Tantra (secret science)
10. Construction of hermitage, temple	10. Destruction of country (war)
11. Planting, gardening	11. Chopping wood, lighting a fire.
12. Building walls, swimming pools, ponds	12. Cutting gems and jewels, sculpting, carpentry
13. Giving charity, lending money	13. Accepting charity, borrowing
14. Marriage, birth of baby	14. Prostitution, sexual indulgence (for male only)

15. Purchasing clothes, ornaments, and land	15. Selling cattle
16. Performing rituals for pacification, appeasement, and attaining worldly prosperity	16. Committing crimes, corrupt practices
17. Friendship, meeting relatives	17. Eradicating, poisoning, or subduing enemies
18. Making efforts to establish peace	18. Hunting, killing, holding a sword
19. Preparing divine medicines or chemicals, practice of alchemy	19. Practicing medicine
20. Treatment of diseases, therapy	20. Fighting, duelling, wrestling, boxing
21. Worshiping of the Guru	21. Seeing a king, meeting and addressing officials
22. Entering a newly constructed house, village, town, new country	22. Driving a vehicle
23. Thinking about a relative's ill health	23. Having a discussion or debate
24. Being initiated into a spiritual order, practicing disciplines	24. Climbing a mountain
25. Addressing one's master	25. Evoking and mastering evil spirits, pacifying poison
26. Service	26. Ordering, giving commands
27. Performing auspicious acts	27. Gambling

28. Starting a new colony order or community	28. Swimming across a torrential river
29. Opening a bank account	29. Worshipping evil spirits, mastering *Mantra* of power, vigour and bravery
30. Knowledge of past, present and future	30. knowledge of unseen and unheard things
31. Curing fever	31. Purification by vomiting, enema, throat cleansing, water purification of the lower intestinal tract, sinus cleansing, Hatha *Yoga* exercises, *Kapal-Bhati*
32. Applying sandal-wood paste to the fore head	32. Using drugs and poisons
33. Tying a four-legged animal	33. Taming or riding a four-legged animal
34. Taking a new vow	34. Drinking liquor
35. Drinkingnon-alcoholic beverages	35. Eating and defecating
36. Urinating	36. Bathing
37. Meditating	37. Captivating members of the opposite sex (for male only) 38. Expressing anger 39. Producing works of illumination 40. Working with accounts, counting preparing ledgers

* Note: The information given in table 2 is very ancient. Although it attempts to span the entire panorama of human activities and behaviour, we can expand upon these lists by observing how modern-day activities fit into the specialised functions of the twin hemispheres (Johari: 1989, p. 27-28).

The *Siva Svarodaya Shastra* strongly suggests undertaking activities, either during the day or night, which are suitable to the dominant nostril. According to *Ayurveda*, *Sushumna* dominance is only meant for calming the system and preparing it for a change in nostrils. It is also said that all plans made during the middle path mode fail—activities started remain incomplete, vows made at this time will be broken and charity becomes useless. Only meditation and other unworldly things are recommended when the middle path operates.

The basic rule regarding the *Siva Svarodaya Shastra* is that a harmony should always be kept between the warm, sun breath flowing through the right nostril, and the cool breath of the left lunar nostril. To give a few examples:

1. During the bright half of the lunar month the Moon rules the night. Therefore, the effects of the Sun are at its minimum. To harmonise this imbalance, it is necessary and advantageous to block the left nostril and allow only the right channel to flow all night.

2. Throughout the dark half of the month, the Moon's influence is absent. During this period it is auspicious to block the Sun channel and let the Moon nostril flow all night.

3. If at any time, and especially when walking or exercising, one feels that the body temperature is suddenly increasing or one feels very tired, block the Sun channel and let the breath flow through the Moon nostril until the tiredness or the heat has gone.

All that has been mentioned here is only a tiny portion of the vast descriptions available in various texts of *Yoga* relating to human nostril operations. My intention in recording at least some of that information is to show how breath is conceived, developed and categorised in terms of different human activities and knowledge. Breath-related knowledge, in my limited reading during the course of this research, seems to be a systematically developed category capable of defining the whole physiological, psychological and spiritual range of human life. Nevertheless, how far the physiological descriptions of the functioning of breath found in this section may be compatible or contradictory in the context of contemporary medicine require further research exploring the ancient medical knowledge against the evidence. Interestingly, the descriptions found in *Marmatherapy* on the growth of the foetus match very well with the meticulous scientific analysis of modern embryology (See section 2.5.1.A. below). Unlike *Ayurveda*, *Marmatherapy* as a system of medical practice is almost unknown to the scholarship and experimental research of contemporary medicine firstly because of the antiquity and exclusiveness of the practice. The second reason for this is that no single authentic text of this traditional medical practice has neither been found nor been translated: this system of knowledge is pronounced in palm leaf manuscripts and exclusively practiced by few traditional families in Southern Travancore. I am aware of the fact that the physiology of breathing found within the traditional metaphoric medical language needs to be balanced against evidence brought out through contemporary medical research, which is not the focus of the thesis. So, in the following section, I will look at some practical approaches to breathing which is central to the line of investigation carried out in this study.

E. Practicing *Svara-Udaya*

Siva Svarodaya Shastra systematically explains the physiological, psychological and spiritual connections between the body and breath. It also suggests a practice known as *Soham Sadhana*, the practice of *So-ham*. The human respiratory system functions in a bi-polar act of inspiration and expiration. The air driven out of the lungs makes the sound *ham* whereas the inhaled air produces the sound *sah*. These two sounds together make the Sanskrit word *hamsah,* which literally means goose, which is a synonym for the 'Supreme Spirit'. The *ham* sound symbolises the male creative principle of consciousness and is known as the seed-sound of Shiva, the unified consciousness. The *sah* sound represents the female creative principle of energy and is the seed-sound of Sakti, the individual self activated by the flow of breath. When the word *hamsa* is reversed, it spells *soham* in Sanskrit. The word *soham* is made of the following vowels and consonants: s+ o + h+ a+ m. When the consonants 's' and '*h*' are taken away from the word, what remains is '*OM*' which is known as the base sound involved in the first motion of universal creation: all the articulated sounds emerge from this seed sound. *Soham* is created through the act of inspiration and expiration which always remains with a person during all states of consciousness.

The practice of this breathing is described as follows: sit in any comfortable posture, with eyes either closed or open, as convenient. Then breathe in slowly and try to hear the *'so'* sound. If you do not hear any sound in the beginning, try to imagine it. While breathing out the *'ham'* sound can also be heard, imagined or mentally repeated. Care should be taken to see that the breathing is continuous and the *'soham'* is not broken up like a verbal articulation. Do it continuously with a break after 15 to 20 minutes until the sound becomes natural and spontaneous. When the rhythm becomes natural one might feel that the breath has stopped but, according to the direction suggested by the text, this is a good sign to show that the practice has become fruitful. According to the *Siva Svarodaya Shastra,* the *'soham'* is essential to higher levels of human consciousness. The practice of *svara udaya*, also called *soham* breathing, as described above, is essential to experiencing higher levels of consciousness. The only system I have found, in my research that provides a clear understanding of the proper practice described as *soham* is that of the South Indian *Siddha* tradition. I will therefore discuss this approach in the following section.

2.5 Breath and the *Siddha* Tradition

Shivaism, as a philosophical system, is the oldest systematic thought and practice of Indian spirituality and has persisted since the pre-historic time of the archaeological finds of the phallic symbol of the Shiva of the Indus valley civilization. It is thus pre-Vedic and the key elements of Shaivite thought can be found in various strands of Indian philosophy, aesthetics and religion, like *Vedas* and *Upanishads* and leading all the way to *Buddhism.*[46] This is because as a philosophical system, Shivaism spread to all the parts of India and also crossed the frontiers of the country to several regions in central Asia. Central to Shivaism is the worship of Shiva, either in the form of a phallic symbol, which represents the idea of the universal and eternal nature of the manifestation of the self, or in the form of various poses, the epitome of which is the *Dancing Natarāj*. Shiva the dancer is the most popular and elegant, representing the cosmic dance of Shiva while witnessing the dissolution of the universe and its fusion in him. On the other hand, it is rather an iconic representation of a deeper Indian cosmic vision, which also considers the performative nature of cognition in terms of time, space and movement. My intention in this section is to demonstrate the key concepts and practices of a breath-related tradition in South India, an offshoot of the Indian Saivite tradition.

This particular tradition is said to have been established by eighteen *Siddhas*, enlightened beings, in the Tamil language whose origin can be dated back to between 3000 BC and 100 AD. It is, therefore, difficult to calculate the exact period in which the texts were written. The South Indian *Siddha* tradition is part of a larger, pan-Indian *tantric-Yoga* movement that spread throughout South Asia, from Sri Lanka in the South to Tibet in the North, between the seventh and eleventh centuries. The most significant aspect of the South Indian Siddha tradition lies in its consideration of the human body as the locus of philosophical discourse. Medical treatises as well as spiritual treatises in the *Siddha* tradition thus share one basic understanding of the crucial relationship between body, breath and consciousness. *Siddha Yoga* is a non-sectarian spiritual tradition that incorporates various body-related disciplines like martial arts, physiotherapy, *Yoga* and *tantric* rituals, as part of its whole structure of practice. According to Douglas Renfrew Brooks, *Siddha Yoga* cannot be reduced to a canon of textual or oral resources, or a fixed set of religious teachings but it is based on certain practices related to breathing.[47] The distinctive element that makes *Siddha Yoga* different from other schools of *Yoga* is its focus on breath-related practice. Hence, rather than repeating *Siddha Yoga*'s theoretical understanding of the relation between the body, breath and consciousness, I intend to explain the spectrum of its practice.

2.5.1 Texts and Authorship

Three major texts represent almost the entire South Indian *Siddha* school of thought. Those three seminal texts are: 1) The *Marmasāstra Samāhāram*[48] of the sage Agastiya 2) the *Thirumandiram*[49] of Siddhar Thirumoolar and 3) *Siddha Veda*[50] of Swami Sivananda

Paramahamsa. Among these three seminal texts, *Siddha Veda* is a comparatively later publication and the author is the founder of *Siddha Samaja*, the foundation for *Siddha* Yogins. The authorship and period of the other two are uncertain because of the antiquity of the texts. The knowledge of *Marma*[51] is part of Siddha physiotherapy, a medical branch initiated by the sage Agastiya, which is different from *Ayurveda. Marma* means the secret points of the body and *Sastra* means manual. The *Marmasastra*, therefore, is to be considered as a practice-based knowledge of the secret *Marma* points of the body. These points are known as secret points because striking on *Marma* points will bring serious damage to the body, but this knowledge is mainly used to cure the neuro-physical disorders. There are 108 secret points in the body. The *Marmasastra* comprises elaborate descriptions of anatomy including the number, types, structure and functions of bones, nerves and muscles along with references to internal organs like the heart and intestines. Much of the information that this ancient medical system offers to the world matches information available in modern medical science, and several other areas covered in the *Marmasastra* are still unknown to modern medicine. The *Marmasastra* also provides a discussion of the ten kinds of breath and their psycho-physical functions. In a wider context, the *Marmasastra* discusses precisely the interactions between body and breath and their further implications in the formation of human consciousness.

The *Thirumandiram* is known as a classical text on the philosophical discourse of the *Siddha* tradition. The text is an esoteric masterpiece of 3000 verses and explains the characteristics of *yogic* practice based on some exclusive breathing systems. Only in the recent past has this work been made available to the English reading public. The whole treatise is divided into nine books and each book is known as *Tantras.* Siddhar Thirumoolar, the author of the *Thirumandiram* illustrates various functions of breath in the body and further explains different breath-related practices used to achieve *Samadhi*, the highest state of human consciousness, according to *Yoga* philosophy. The intention of Shivananda Paramahamsa in writing *Siddha Veda* was to explain the secrets of *Siddha Yoga*'s particular breathing practices by making them simple and available to laymen who are not able to comprehend them properly because of the confusing and metaphoric language of the classical texts like the

Thirumandiram. In fact, the *Marmasastra* and the *Thirumandiram* share several features in terms of terminology and concepts because medical terms are being used to explain spiritual practices and vice versa.

Like various other ancient Indian texts, the authorship of the *Marmasastra* is unclear and the period in which it was written is also debatable. The sage Agastiya is accountable for the compilation of the treatise. Many of the palm leaf manuscripts of the *Marmasastra* give evidence of the existence of the sage Agastiya as the author because they normally carry the inscription of his name towards the end of the text. He is known as one of the eighteen *Siddha* Yogins in the Sanga period in Tamil literature between B.C.3000 and A.D.100. *Tholkappiyam,* the oldest available text in the Tamil language, which is dated between B.C.1000 and B.C.300, refers to Sage Agastiya as one who lives in the mountains of the Southern range. This clearly gives some idea about his period as it is before *Tholkappiyam* was written. It is also important to note that, in a later period, exactly the same reference to Agastiya could be found in the epic *Ramayana*, which was written in approximately B.C.400. Considering this limited textual evidence we can assume that the *Marmasastra* was written somewhere between B.C.3000 and B.C.1000, which might perhaps be concurrent with Vedic literature or even before the existence of *Rig Veda* if the calculations are historically accurate. But there are problems in accurately locating the period of these ancient texts because of their pre-historic origins. In contrast, the period of the *Thirumandiram* is exactly calculated between 5 A.D and 6 A.D though there is nothing much left as far as the biographical details of the author are concerned, except a few references that are found in other ancient literary works in Tamil. The following section will discuss the *Marmasastra's* understanding of the human embodiment and the breath's crucial role in it.

A. The Body in the *Marmasastra*

The *Marmasastra* viewed the human body as a manifest phenomenon. In order to explain the genesis of human embodiment, Agastiya, the author of the *Marmasastra,* begins with the unmanifest, the timeless reality, from which the physicality of individual existence becomes manifest. The body as the physical manifestation of various natural principles and qualities is further analysed in detail in terms of the anatomical structure of the body. In this way, considering the human body as the material manifestation of 'pure existence', the *Marmasastra* proposes an important idea about the body—that it is the only available medium to experience and understand 'timeless reality' since the body is part of that pure universal substance. Agastiya, in this context, clearly says that the presence of breath in the body is the way in which 'timeless reality' can be grasped, and hence the *Marmasastra* provides further clarifications about the inter-dynamic relationship between the body and breath. On the whole the *Marmasastra* includes meticulous descriptions about the metaphysical, physiological and psychophysical viewpoints of the body.

The process of the genesis of the human body in the therapeutic discourse of the *Marmasastra* is presented through twenty five verses of the invocatory preamble in the form of a small book called *Brahmanila Sutram.*[52] These verses include the metaphysical view of the body, the ethics of a Marma practitioner and the origin and elementary components of body. The *jiva*, the embodiment, is created out of *Brahman*, the unmanifest. The *Marmasastra* explains this metaphysical origin by using two terms: *para* and *apara*. The first is known as the underlying potential energy of the manifest world, whereas the second is explained as the individual knowing self or the manifest. The origin involves a split—that of the essential nature of the individual taking shape from the essential source of all manifestations. All manifestations, including individual beings, have a form of identity and this identity is limited in the sense that it is manifested from the unlimited unmanifest. Thus the individual being is placed in a definite time and space through this manifestation and separated from its awareness of the totality of being, the substratum of individual existence. Hence, individual existence is part of a whole and thus the relationship between the manifest individual and the unmanifest, unconditioned and timeless reality is that of identity and difference. Agastiya says that the ignorance of a universal totality relating to individual existence is inherited in the genesis of the body (M.S:I: I: 1-4).[53] This ignorance causes duality between the knowing self (*jiva*) and the timeless reality, the substratum of the universe. The knowing individual self, the *jiva*, is activated through *Prāna,* the life force, through nostril operations. Breath causes the emergence of the knowing self. It also functions as the reason for the unawareness of the relations between unconditioned universal reality and individual existence. Agastiya further explains that through the union of *para* and *apara,* the union of *jiva* and *brahman*, the union of breath and consciousness, the fundamental ignorance involved in the nature of individual being can be eliminated (M.S: I: II: 1-4).[54] Agastiya suggests a breath-related practice in order to eliminate this ignorance and to achieve that state of human consciousness that is known as the highest state of *Samadhi* in various Shaivite traditions. It is also known as the unified state according to the Vedanta model of consciousness.

There are four recurrent images in the *Marmasastra* about the human body: the landscape, the tree, the house and the cosmos. The body as landscape contains thousands and thousands of rivers in the form of blood vessels that spring from the pool of the heart, where the eternal tree is planted with plentiful roots of nerves spreading deeply all over the body whose trunk is the spine that carries the immortal flower of the thousand-petalled lotus on the top (M.S: 1:4).[55] The name of the tree is *sushumna*, the vital nerve running through inside the vertebral column starting from the bottom of the spine and terminating in the brain. The other two major nerves, called *Ida* and *Pingala*, follow *sushumna,* running from the same source at the bottom of the spine on the exterior through both sides of the spine. These three major nerves are called three *Nadis*, the vital channels of the subtle body, which are connected to nostril operations.

According to the view of *Marmasāstra,* the body emerges out of the primary natural elements like earth, water, fire, ether and air. The body is again divided into the three zones of Sun, Moon and Fire. Each zone is connected to the system of breathing and the left and right nostrils of the body. For instance, the left nostril is the Moon zone, which is connected to the left *Nadi* called *Ida,* and the right nostril is the Sun zone, which is connected to the right *Nadi* called *Pingala.* The fire zone of the body is related to the *Nadi* called *Sushumna.* This *Nadi* runs inside the spine and is connected to the middle of the nasal cycle. This middle nostril path is crucial to *yogic* techniques of breathing because several intricate and exclusive techniques of breathing are connected to this middle path. As I mentioned in my discussion of the *Siva Svarodaya Shastra*, according to the *Marmasastra*, a healthy body normally breaths 21,600 times within 24 hours and natural breathing changes from left to right and right to left perpetually and intermittently in its course during the 24 hours. In each changeover from left to right and right to left, breath flows through both nostrils. This particular nostril operation is called the middle path. I will discuss the importance of this middle path breathing in the following sections. The *Marmasastra* and *Siva Svarodaya Shastra* share similar understandings of the nature and inner dynamics of breath in the body. We see that breath has been incorporated in various disciplines from classical Indian music to *Ayurveda, Marma, Upanishads, Sāmkhya* and *Yoga*. Breath is perhaps the one underlying common element to all these disciplines.

The metaphoric image of the body as cosmos is connected to the three distinctive modes of nostril operations: the left, the right and the middle. The left nostril is metaphorically considered as the Moon where as the right is known as the Sun. Human respiration consists of the constant interplay or the changeover between left and right nostrils, and the *Marmasastra* metaphorically emphasises that the Sun and the Moon rise and set several times in the cosmologic orbits in the body (M.S: 1:5).[56] This nasal cycle of the rise and fall of Sun and Moon indicates the passage of time in the body and in our consciousness. All the daily activities of the body and all the daily senses of our consciousness are interconnected to the temporal aspects of left and right nostril modes. The middle path suggests a timeless sense of consciousness which I will discuss in the fourth chapter, in terms of breath and consciousness. Another metaphoric image of the body as the house is connected to the structural pattern of the subtle body. In the *Marmasastra,* the body is divided vertically from the bottom of the spine to the crown of the head into six sections and each of these sections contains one vital energy centre, which is known as the psychophysical centre of the body. These psychophysical body centres are called *Cakras* and both *Yoga* as well as *tantric* traditions provide knowledge about the existence of these centres in the body. As we saw in the earlier sections of the *Sangitaratnakara of Sarangadeva,* the *Cakras* function as the centres of consciousness at various planes situated between the anus and the crown at the top of the head. Concentration on and control of one or many of these centres bestows enormous psychophysical powers. According to most of the *yogic* systems, the aim of practising *Yoga* is to train the mind to concentrate upon and penetrate through all these centres in order to achieve a complete mastery over the physical and the psychic body. The aim is also said to be to attain freedom from the limited perception of mind and matter. However, this structure of the psychophysical body has nine doors according to the *Marmasastra*: two eyes, two ears, two nostrils, two inner throats and one mouth. In this house lives the person who records each perception, sound, smell, touch and experience and there also lives another person on a higher level who witnesses the person who is recording all the accounts. Even from this initial observation, the body, mind and the consciousness of human embodiment, as illustrated by the *Marmasastra* are inseparably interconnected and the role of breath connecting all these physiological, psychological and metaphysical elements is clearly established in its therapeutic discourse. The *Marmasastra* shows the body as a labyrinth: the labyrinth of breath.

Both in *Marmasāstra* and in the *Thirumandiram* the origin and growth of the foetus is explained elaborately and, in the seventh Tantra of the *Thirumandiram*, Thirumoolar states that life span, death and diseases, intelligence and the overall health and well-being of the human organism will be defined by the nature of their sexual copulation and the quality and positions of their breathing (7:20:1079-80).[57] The movement and dynamism of male breath is the only force that brings the seminal fluid to the interiority of the womb. In *Marmasāstra*, the growth of the foetus is calculated on a weekly basis as is the case with modern medical embryology. According to *Marmasāstra*, fertilization occurs in a flower-like region within the internal system where the female and the male gametes fuse; the pictorial illustration of the ampullary region of the uterine tube in modern embryology shows the ampulla region as having the shape of a flower. Even more similarities between *Marmasāstra* and modern embryology could be traced through this comparison. The growth of the foetus is given in detail in *Marmasāstra*. The first nine days are described day by day. On the first day the size of the foetus is a small grain of mustard seed and on the fourth day it becomes the size of a coriander seed and finally, on the seventh day, the size of a small lemon (MS: IV:12-13).[58] Interestingly, the movement of the male sperm is mentioned in *Marmasāstra* in relation to the entrance of a certain length of breath in the uterus.

As *Marmasāstra* describes the process, breath is incorporated at the very earliest stage of fertilization and helps the formation of foetus (MS: IV: 12).[59] In this sense, *Marmasāstra* proposes the internalization of breath in the foetus at an early stage of its formation. It also clearly says that miscarriage can take place as a result of improper initiation of breath. As Agastiya goes on, in the first week the natural elements like fire and water split apart and form into adequate combinations and in the second week the basic form of the foetus changes from spherical to oval. According to the language of *Marmasāstra*, the foetus will take the shape of a plantain flower. Followed by this, the neck forms in the second week roughly separating the body from the head and consequently in the third and fourth weeks the head figures distinctively. The body is shaped like a spoon in the fifth week including the formation of legs, hands and the fingers. The 72,000 nerves emerge and spread all over the body in the sixth and the seventh weeks. In the eighth week pulsation begins and thus movement takes place. This is the time when the foetus consumes liquid food through the umbilical cord and the body grows further as a result of this. Finally, Agastiya says, in the ninth week, the crown of the head is covered with soft layer of bone and skin and this is followed by the activating of the brain and the bodily senses. According to Agastiya, the covering of this soft layer of bone over the crown and the emergence of intelligence in the body are related. The emergence of the intelligence and the bodily senses, according to Agastiya, prevents it from knowing the origin (MS:4:13,14,15).[60] For Agastiya, the growth of the foetus is complete by the ninth week and he does not say anything about the further growth from there onwards. In my comparative reading of both *Marmasāstra* and modern embryology, I can see several similarities between these two medical traditions in terms of the origin of the human body. Agastiya says that the genesis of the body and the 'internalisation of breath' in the foetus are inseparable and hence he draws the following conclusions (MS: I: 3-10)[61]:

1. The body is the manifestation of the primordial energy mediated by breath.

2. The quality and the mode of operation of the male and female breath determine the health and destiny of the foetus.

3. The internalised breath activates in the pre-born body, which flows out through the nostrils during birth and hence the baby breathes in, which is the first autonomous individual act.
4. The act of breathing creates individual consciousness and the most important knowledge to learn from the teacher is to internalize the breath in order to experience *turiya*. The term *turiya* refers to alteration of consciousness which goes beyond the daily consciousness.

From another perspective, Thirumoolar explains the role of breath further in the formation and growth of the foetus since the pattern and direction of the breathing of the male and female participants in the sexual act define the destiny of the human body. The length of the breath at the time when the orgasm occurs defines the life span of the child. If it is 5 *vara*,[62] the life span will be 100 years, whereas if it is reduced to 4 *Vara*, the life span will be 80 years: one who knows the path of true *Yoga* can control destiny(TM:2:271). Moreover, the male child will be born if the operating nostril is right at the time of sexual copulation and a female child if it is left. There will be twin children if *Apana*, one among the ten forms of breath in the body, dominates. (TM: 2: 274 - 5).[63]

Both *Marmasāstra* and the *Thirumandiram* share the understanding of the relation between the body, breath and consciousness. According to both these systems, there is a split involved in the origin. Nostril operation through birth creates this split between individual consciousness and the non-dual state of unified consciousness. Therefore, the unified state of consciousness can be regained only through internalising individual respiration. Both Agastiya and Thirumoolar suggest that internalisation of breathing is a technique through which the breath can be brought back to its natural location. According to Thirumoolar, the act of internalising respiration initially evokes vital psychophysical energy in the body and then an extended system of practice will enable the individual to attain the sense of a unified state of consciousness, *Samadhi* (II Tantra: 203). Agastiya further clarifies the existence of a cave-like place inside the human skull and says that the act of the internalisation of breath involves the careful utilisation of this cave. In the *Marmasastra,* this place is known as the "cave of colours". In my understanding, the *Siddha* system of breathing techniques is based on two ideas: 1) Agastiya's cave 2) the internalisation of breath. I will explain these ideas further in the following sections.

B. *Marma* and the Body

What is Marma? How many *Marma* points are there in the body? What are their effects in the body? As Agastiya explains, marmas are the junctions, knots and ends of *Nadis* where *prana*, the life force, is present. Any serious pressure or blow at these points will seriously affect the life span of the system (MS:II: 30).[64] *Marmasāstra* offers treatments and medicines for any fatal afflictions of the body through a systematic practice relating to the *Marma* points. Marma points are categorised into two sections:

1) 12 most fatal points. If hit in specific ways, death will be immediate.

2) 96 fatal points. If hit, death will not be immediate but the impact will create various disorders in the system.

Marmasāstra elaborately discusses the locations of *Marma* points in the body including the directions and measures to locate those places properly. The *thilasakala*, for instance, is an important *Marma* is located by the side of the upper portion of the eyes, exactly ½ an inch (*nellida*) down from the centre of the eyebrows (MS: II: 40).[65] Agastiya further explains the ways of attacking the *Marma* point as well as treating the body once a *Marma* point has been hit. Kaimanan Karunakaran Vaidyar lists the names of all the 108 *Marma* points and further describes the physical signs that appear when any one of them has been hit, and the way to treat the effects.[66] To give an example, *Malar Marma* can be applied in the following manner in a fight: block the enemy's right hand blow by your left hand while taking a martial position, keeping your left leg in front, and then use your stretched and focused right palm to hit the *Marma* spot. The pressure should be calculated properly in order to create the full effect that is possible in relation to this particular *Marma* point. The middle finger of the right palm is pushed one inch (*ira)* inside on the *Marma* spot and then dragged downwards with appropriate pressure. This is the proper direction of attack on that *Marma*. Both the hands and the legs of the enemy will be paralysed as a result of hitting this particular *Marma* in this particular way.

Though Agastiya explains the treatment elaborately, he requests again and again that no one should attack on this *Marma* in order to destroy the body. It is very important to note that Agastiya explains all the marmas for eliminating the physical disorders of the body through treatment, but not for damaging the body. According to Agastiya, only a mature person has the right to know and practice this secret knowledge of the body. He should also have the quality of a yogi who can control the emotions and worldly desires (MS: I: 2).[67] Each *Marma* point is the location in the body where breath stays and any form of blow on those points will create disorder in the function of breath in the body. Hence, Marma is the physical point of the dynamics of breath functioning in the body.

2.5.2 Agastiya's Cave

Agastiya explains the existence of a cave situated at the base of the palate region behind the uvula when he demonstrates a breath-related practice in the context of the unified state of consciousness. This centre is the most important region in the body in both Siddha *Yoga* in general and the *Marmasastra* in particular. According to Agastiya, breath has to be retained concealed in this cave in order to attain the highest level of human consciousness. Perception and experiences of the body will change when the breath is concealed in this cave. As Agastiya explains the method, breath has to be pushed through the middle path at the time when both 'doors open'. Here, the doors indicate both left and right nostrils and when both the left and the right nostrils are open that is the middle path. Pushing the breath towards the *cave* through the middle path is thus the practice suggested by Agastiya to internalise breathing. Breathing at this stage will be through *ul-mulam,* the single internal nostril leading to the *panchavarna-guha,* the cave of five colours (MS: II: 211-219).[68] The *Marmasastra* does not provide any further explanation of the five colours in relation to the cave. Nevertheless, the description of the breath-related practice presented in the *Marmasastra* is the core practice of the South Indian Siva tradition which is preserved in *Siddha Yoga* as *Siddha Vidya.*

2.5.3 *Siddha Vidya*

Yoga is understood as the union of two forces and several interpretations of it explain these forces differently as individual self and higher levels of consciousness, mind and higher levels of consciousness and so on but *Siddha Yoga* clearly says that the union is the union of two forms of breath: *prana* and *apana.* The practice suggested by the *Marmasastra* clearly focuses on this idea of the union of the bi-polar movement of breath. This Siddha practice is further explained in the *Thirumandiram* as: the union is the fusion of Sun and Moon into one at the upper portion of the nostrils beyond the uvula.[69] The Sun and Moon here suggest the right and left nostril modes and the practitioner is requested to wake up early in the morning at dawn and then practice the internalisation through the middle path while combining Sun and Moon, the two operating nostrils, into one. Swami Sivananda Paramahamsa further explains the practice as the union of the bi-polar movement of breathing. As he elucidates it, *prana* is the breath that stays in and *apana* is the breath that flows out. And the *Siddha Vidya* is the knowledge of combining the *apana* with *prana* without allowing the *apana* to flow out. *Siddha Vidya,* in this sense, redirects the outward flow into the proper internal channels (See Chapter four).[70] A further special instruction is given by Paramahamsa: breath needs to be prolonged and directed upwards in this process as a bellows emits a stream of air used for blowing air into a fire.

In my field research in Kerala, I have identified twenty-four patterns of sequential breathing known as *Gati,* which literally means directions. This system offers twenty-four patterns of breath directions consisting mostly of the sounds of birds and animals, which vibrate in different parts of the body. Out of these twenty-four patterns, eighteen are to do with a convenient sitting position and the remaining six are to do with bodily movements. All twenty-four patterns are intended to create very high energy levels in the body. Both *Siddha Vidya* and *Gati* are breath-related practices clearly understood and practised by people who belong to *Siddha* lineage.

Summary

Several concepts on and approaches to breath illustrated in this Chapter clearly show the importance of the dynamics of breath in the entire psychophysical existence of the human organism. Breath is the basic substance of the physical body, which activates all its physical functions. Mind is something which is realised in the body and hence all mental movements have corresponding breathing patterns. As we have seen, several traditions, Aristotle, *Tao, Sāmkhya*, the *Upanishads*, *Yoga*, *Ayurveda*, Classical music, the *Marmasastra* and the *Siddha Veda*, consider and establish the connection between breath and consciousness and there are systems available to alter the sense of consciousness through specific practices related to breathing. *Soham* and *Siddha Vidya* are the most reliable practices available in this context. The following are the ideas derived from this Chapter:

1. Breath is considered as the most important physical, psychological and spiritual category in Indian traditions in general and in the South Indian *Siddha* tradition, in particular.

2. Breath-related methods exist in *Yoga* to explore the dynamics of breath in the body in order to enhance the psycho-physical energy level.

3. The *Siva Svarodaya Shastra,* the *Sangitaratnakara,* the *Marmasastra* and the *Siddha Veda* refer to three modes of nostril operations, which are left, right and the middle path. These texts also suggest that left and right path breathing relate to a conventional sense of time whereas the middle path suggests a shift in the daily sense of time in the direction of an altered state of consciousness.

4. Practices like *Soham* and *Siddha Vidya* show the implications of the middle path breathing in terms of altered states of consciousness gained through systematic practice.

5. The link between the nostril operations and the shift of the sense of time is the most important idea derived from this chapter because both the philosophy and practice of the nostrils similarly indicate the element of temporality involved in nostril operations.

The emphasis on the middle path breathing in terms of temporality, emotion and consciousness will be discussed further in the following chapters. What middle path breathing is and how it is connected to a shift in our daily sense of time, and how temporality relates to our meaning and consciousness are the questions this thesis is going to address in the following Chapters. In the next chapter I intend to look at the implications of breath on theatre training and performance, both traditional and modern, and Eastern and Western.

Notes

[1] Aristotle, *Aristotle on the Soul: Prava Naturalia, On breath*, tr: Hett. W.S, (London: William Heinemann Ltd & Harvard University Press, 1936), pp. 484-517.
[2] Ibid., p. 484.
[3] Ibid., p. 485.
[4] Ibid., p. 503.
[5] Ibid., p. 401.
[6] Ibid., p. 489.
[7] Ibid., p. 29.
[8] Paul Wildish., *The Book of Ch'i*, (Boston: Journey Editions, 2000), p. 22 .
[9] Ibid., p. 23.
[10] Ibid., p. 24.
[11] Ibid., p. 32-33.
[12] Gerald James Larson and Ram Shankar Bhattacharya, (ed.), *Sāmkhya: A Dualist Tradition in Indian Philosophy*, (Princeton: Princeton University Press, 1987), 51.
[13] Wilhelm Halbfass, "*Space or Matter: The Concept of Akāsa in Indian Thought*", Rabindranath Tagore Lecture, Centre for Philosophy and Foundations of Science, New Delhi, 1999.
[14] See footnote 45 below for further details on Saivism.
[15] Surendranath Dasgupta, *A History of Indian Philosophy,* Vol. 5 (Cambridge: Cambridge University Press, 1955), 81.
[16] Pulinbihari Chakravarti, *Origin and Development of the Sāmkhya System of Thought,* (London: Luzac & Co, Ltd, 1975) p. 255.
[17] Ibid., p. 256.
[18] Ibid., p. 256.
[19] Ibid., p. 120.
[20] Ibid., p. 257.
[21] See for details. Ibid., p. 265-66. The enumeration of the five breaths seems to be different in South Indian Siddha tradition because Agastiya and Thirumular listed ten breaths instead of five.
[22] Swami Prabhavananda and Frederick Manchester, *The Upanishads: Breath of the Eternal,* (California: Vedanta Press, 1971) p. xvii.
[23] Fritjof Capra, *The Tao of Physics,* (London: Fontana/Collins, 1981) p. 93-96.
[24] Ibid., p. 95.
[25] Ralph Yarrow, *Indian Theatre: Theatre of Origin, Theatre of Freedom,* (London: Curzon, 2001), p. 9-10.
[26] Ibid., p. 9-10.
[27] Daniel Meyer Dinkgräfe, *Approaches to Acting: Past and Present,* (London & New York: Continuum, 2001), p. 95.
[28] Ibid., p. 95.
[29] Sir John Woodroffe, *The Garland of Letters*, (Madras: Ganesh & Co, 2001), p. 228
[30] Ibid., p. 232.
[31] Mircea Eliade, *Yoga: Immortality and Freedom,* (tr. Willard R. Trask), (Princeton: Princeton University Press, 1969), p. 3.
[32] Ibid., p. 7.

[33] Ibid., p. 47.
[34] B.S.K Iyengar, *Light on Yoga*, (New Delhi: Harper Collins, 2000) p. 37.
[35] Yogi Ramacharaka, *Science of Breath,* (London: Fowler, 1960) p. 28-32.
[36] Dhirendra Brahmachari, *Yogic Suksma Vyayama,* (New Delhi: Dhirendra *Yoga* Publications, 1956), p. xxii.
[37] R. K. Shringy and Prem Lata Sharma, *Sangitaratnakara of Sarngadeva,* (tr.) vol. 1, (New Delhi: Munshiram Manoharlal, 1991), p. 85-6.
[38] See for details. Sir John Woodroffe, *The Garland of Letters,* (Madras: Genesh & co, 2001), p. 276.
[39] R. K. Shringy and Prem Lata Sharma, *Sangitaratnakara of Sarngadeva,* (tr.) vol. 1, (New Delhi: Munshiram Manoharlal, 1991), p. 99.
[40] Swami Sivapriyananda, *Secret Power of Tantrik Breathing,* (New Delhi: Abhinav Publications, 1996) p. 3.
[41] Harish Johari, *Breath, Mind and Consciousness,*(Rochester & Vermont: Destiny Books, 1989), p. 2-3.
[42] Ibid., p. 11-15.
[43] Ibid., p. 14-16.
[44] Ibid., p. 17.
[45] Swami Sivapriyananda, *Secret Power of Tantrik Breathing,* (New Delhi: Abhinav Publications, 1996) p. 24.
[46] In *An outline of history of Saiva Philosophy*, Kanti Chandra Pandey briefly discusses the deep and extensive influence of Shivaism to various other philosophical and religious systems. As he points out, in Rig*veda*, there are verses, which refer to *Rudra,* another name of Shiva. In *Sāmaveda*, there are also hymns addressed to *Rudra.* Whereas in *Yajurveda*, the name of *Rudra* is mentioned among other names of the Gods in the Section XVI of the *Vājasaneya Samhitā* and in the *Taittiriya Samhitā* of *Yajurveda* section IV, 5. In the *Atharvaveda*, for instance, there are many collections of hymns worshipping Shiva mainly in VI, XI and XV sections and therefore, K.C. Pandey argues that *Shivaism* as a philosophical system has deeply influenced Vedic and post-Vedic systems of thought and spiritual practice though it never shows an unbroken continuity in the Indian religio-philosophic traditions. Buddha refers to *Shivaism* in his own way as *Shiva Vijjā*, which is later on interpreted as *Bhūta Vijjā*, or exorcism by Buddhaghoṣa a 5th A. D commentator of Buddhism (K.C. Pandey, 1999: 1-3). K.C. Pandey illustrates briefly the debates between Buddhism and monistic Shivaism of Kashmir while explaining Abhinavagupta's refutation of Buddha's negation of the unified Subject proposed by Shaivite School. Buddha does not admit the existence of any kind of permanent subject, individual or universal but being for Buddha is rather a series of momentary being. Utpalācārya and Abhinavagupta reassess this Buddhist notion of momentary being against the philosophical background of non-dualist Shivaism as the synthesis of experience is not possible on the basis of Buddha's views of momentariness of subject. Besides underpinning the most predominant limitation in Buddhist epistemology in terms of cognition and the objective relationship of the knower, monistic Shaivite School explores the epistemic basis of Shiva metaphysics while explaining the foundational inter relations of memory and differentiation in cognition (K.C. Pandey, 1999: 195-206)

[47] Douglas Renfrew Brooks, *Meditation Revolution: A History and Theology of the Siddha Yoga Lineage,* (ed.), (New Delhi: Motilal Banarsidass, 2000), p. xxiv.
[48] KanjiramKulam K. Kochukrishnan Nadar, *Marmasastra Samāhāram*, Deshabhivardhini Publishing House, Trivandrum: 1968.
[49] Thiruvallam Bhaskaran Nair, *Thirumandiram Moovariram* (Mal.), Kerala Vidya Peth, Trivandrum: 1976.
[50] Swami Shivananda Paramahamsar, *Siddha Veda* (Mal), Siddha Samagam, Vadakara (Kerala): 1922.
[51] My understanding of this secret system of knowledge related to the secret points of the body is largely derived initially from my own family tradition through the practice of martial arts, physiotherapy. Secondly, it derives from textual sources. Apparently, the information about this knowledge has mainly resided in palm leaf manuscripts and preserved by individual families who are traditionally authorised to practice. Most of these families are situated in the extreme Southern regions of old Travancore, which is a district, called Kanyakumari, of Tamil Nadu. I myself posess couple of palm leaf manuscripts as part of my family tradition.
[52] KanjiramKulam K. Kochukrishnan Nadar, *Marmasastra Samāhāram*, (Trivandrum: Deshabhivardhini Publishing House, 1968), p. 1-4.
[53] Ibid., p.1-4.
[54] Ibid., p. 1-4.
[55] Ibid., p. 4.
[56] Ibid., p. 4 –5.
[57] Thiruvallam Balakrishnan Nair, *Thirumantram Moovayiram*, (Trivandrum: Vijnana-bhavan Printers, 1976), p. 219. A translation of *Thirumantiram* appeared in Malayam, the regional language of Kerala and I use this edition for my references.
[58] KanjiramKulam K. Kochukrishnan Nadar, *Marmasastra Samāhāram*, (Trivandrum: Deshabhivardhini Publishing House, 1968), p. 148.
[59] Ibid., p. 148.
[60] Ibid., pp. 148-149.
[61] Ibid., p. 4 -6.
[62] It is an ancient unit of measure, which is no longer in use.
[63] Thiruvallam Balakrishnan Nair, *Thirumantram Moovayiram*, (Trivandrum: Vijnanabhavan Printers, 1976) p. 76.
[64] KanjiramKulam K. Kochukrishnan Nadar, *Marmasastra Samāhāram*, (Trivandrum: Deshabhivardhini Publishing House, 1968), p. 20.
[65] Ibid., p. 22.
[66] Kaimanam Karunakaran Vaidyar, *Marmasastra Patangal,* (Trivandrum: Published by the author, 2002), p. 49.
[67] KanjiramKulam K. Kochukrishnan Nadar, *Marmasastra Samāhāram*, (Trivandrum: Deshabhivardhini Publishing House, 1968), p. 2.
[68] Ibid., p. 51-52.
[69] Thiruvallam Balakrishnan Nair, *Thirumantram Moovayiram*, (Trivandrum: Vijnanabhavan Printers, 1976) p. 181.
[70] Swami Shivananda Paramahamsar, *Siddha Veda* (Mal), Siddha Samagam, Vadakara (Kerala): 1922. p. 95.

Chapter Three
Breath: Training and Performance

Meyer-Dinkgräfe investigates the world-wide origins of acting to assert that the origin of acting is "concerned with fundamental characteristics of human nature": myth and ritual, storytelling, imitation and a gift for fantasy,[1] which are mainly found in pre-modern traditions of performance across the world. Storytelling, for instance, is an ancient art of narrating "an event, real or imagined, presented by a narrator" who takes various roles in the story as and when it is required. According to Meyer-Dinkgräfe, theatre has developed from storytelling: individual members of a group shared impersonation of the story's characters. Similarly, rituals are used to indicate the glory of supernatural powers or local heroes. Rituals often include some form of music, dance, speech, masks and costumes, as does theatre. Meyer-Dinkgräfe emphasises that though societies abandon their rituals in the course of their social development, the stories, myths and rituals remain as part of the worldwide origin of theatre. The Vedic rituals described in the *Natyasastra* and the two mythical stories of Japanese theatre, the first actor Umihiko and the Sun-goddess, clearly show the validity of the argument that the worldwide origin of theatre has a strong ritual base.[2] The *Natyasastra* and the Japanese mythical stories, according to Meyer-Dinkgräfe, offer the preliminary information that actors need to be "immensely skilled, suggesting a demanding training".[3]

Actor training has a long tradition in Eastern forms of theatre, whereas in the West that tradition is comparatively shorter. In the introduction to her anthology of essays on 20th century actor training, Hodge offers an extensive account of a range of concepts and practical models proposed by the most well-known Western actor trainers, many of which are indebted to Eastern models of actor training. *Noh* theatre, which dates back to fifteenth century Japan and *Kathakali*, the dance theatre of South India, which evolved around the same period, for instance, have systematic methods of training the actor's psycho-physicality. Western approaches to training, though they developed properly as a systematic canon only as late as the twentieth century, nevertheless provide a rich spectrum of meaningful concepts, assumptions and ideas and practice. Konstantin Stanislavsky,

Vsevolod Meyerhold, Michael Chekhov and Jacques Copeau are considered the early pioneers among twentieth century actor trainers in the West. A further list of director/actor trainers in Western Europe and Northern America vividly shows the richness of the tradition: Bertolt Brecht, Joan Littlewood, Lee Strasberg, Stella Adler and Joseph Chaikin, Jacques Lecoq, Jerzy Grotowski, Peter Brook and Eugenio Barba. All of them have remarkably influenced the development of Western theatre by addressing issues relating to the actor's mind/body dynamics, the actor-spectator relationship and spatial and temporal dimensions relating to the body and theatrical experience. The investigations put forward by all of these practitioners were based on understanding and training the fundamental psycho-physical elements involved in the actor's art. As a result of this, a variety of terms and concepts have developed throughout the century, which clearly indicate the practitioners' intention or approach to theatre in general and acting in particular: Artaud's *cruelty,* Brook's *total* and *holy* theatres, Grotowski's *translumination,* and Barba's *presence* are only the most important examples. According to Hodge, the widening influence of objective scientific research at the turn of the 19th to the 20th century, particularly the psychological exploration of the subconscious mind, and the growing awareness of the rigorous training in Eastern traditions are the two major sources of inspiration to Western actor training (Hodge 2000, 2).

Hodge identifies two aspects essential to actor training in the West: availability of performance material mostly from the East through intercultural exchanges, and the explosion of knowledge, particularly the systematic methods of psychoanalysis and anthropological theories. While investigating the ancient roots of actor training Meyer-Dinkgräfe suggests three key elements fundamental to Eastern training: religious in function, ritual in practice and spiritual in purpose. Western training is embedded more into an analytical and intercultural tradition whereas the focus of the Eastern training is more ritualistic and spiritual in nature. Meyer-Dinkgräfe's views require further exploration in the context of contemporary actor training investigating how spiritual and ritual aspects are important in training the mind and the body of the actor, and how they work as a method. Citing from Meyer-Dinkgräfe, "Meyerhold placed much emphasis on the actor's physical training and discipline" by developing a set of psychophysical exercises called *biomechanics.* Biomechanics incorporated elements of acrobatics and gymnastics including some more complex exercises like *études* which enable the actor to be more responsive to the sequences of his action, in the sense that each turn, halt and lean back is crucially important to make the action 'throwing the stone' more convincing. Grotowski developed a training method that enables his actors to reach that state of mind he called *translumination*, which according to him is something "achieving a state of sacred theatre, in which spontaneity and discipline co-exist and mutually reinforce each other".[4] For Brook, actor training initially implies physical training leading to a body that is "open, responsive, and unified in all its responses", and secondly, training the emotions, leading to the actor's "capacity to feel". For Barba, "training is a process of self-definition, a process of self-discipline", and therefore, "training is outwardly physical".

This chapter analyses how breath has been integrated in training and performance of traditional Eastern as well as the contemporary Western theatres. The chapter is divided into two major sections in which traditional Eastern and contemporary Western actor training will be discussed in terms of how breath has been integrated into practice. In the Eastern section I am mainly focusing on Keralan performance traditions, with particular emphasis on *Kudiyattam*, the Sanskrit theatre of India, mainly because I am familiar with this tradition and also have access to the material available locally. *Kudiyattam* is a highly stylised theatrical form with a strong emphasis on many years of systematic and complex training methods. Other areas of discussion in the same section will draw on the *Natyasastra*, the theatre manual describing the Indian concept of training and performance, with special emphasis on the concept of *rasa. Rasa* is the delight or bliss experienced by the audience as the result of a theatrical event. It emerges from the interaction between stage and audience. The *Natyasastra* describes eight *rasas* (later commentaries add a ninth) and provides detailed instructions as to how the actor can achieve the experience of any one *rasa* in the spectator.

In the section on contemporary Western actor training I shall focus mainly on the 20th century. Artaud does not create a practical training method, but we see accounts of some systems based on breath in his writings. I will refer to these as they become relevant in my discussions of the role breath plays in the theory and practice of Copeau, Stanislavski, Grotowski and Lecoq. I shall also look at some recent approaches like John Martin's intercultural training, Phillip Zarrilli's training method based on *Kalarippayattu* and Susanna Bloch's Alba Emoting, demonstrating how the understanding of breath has changed in the 21st century. Two further sub-sections will deal with the relation of breath and voice in the work of Cecily Berry and Catherine Fitzmaurice, and theoretical understanding of breath presented by Malekin, Yarrow and Meyer-Dinkgräfe in their various critical writings that consider breath as a potential ingredient in actor training in the context of consciousness in training and performance.

3.1 Breath in Eastern Actor Training

In this section of chapter three I want to explore to what extent the knowledge available in the Indian disciplines and texts of *Yoga*, *Ayurveda* and the *Marmasastra*, has been incorporated in the practices of actor training. In particular, in the context of the thesis, I am interested in the extent to which the knowledge about breath found in these Indian disciplines and texts forms part of actor training. In this discussion I focus on performance traditions of Kerala, for two reasons. Firstly, as I am from Kerala, I am most familiar with the performance traditions of that region of India. Secondly the performance tradition in Kerala is inter-disciplinary in nature in the sense that it combines knowledge and practice from traditions such as martial arts, medicine and meditation. The repertoire of performance in Kerala has been developed through centuries of careful experiments, renovations and restorations informed by other systems of knowledge.[5] The tradition of martial arts is not merely "holding weapons and engaging in combats" rather it represents "a composite culture incorporating elements from the whole range of people's social, religious, artistic and cultural life".[6] Several martial arts traditions in Kerala including *Kalarippayattu* have a legendary origin and influenced deeply the development of *Kathakali* and other performance forms. Similarly, traditional medical knowledge of *Ayurveda* and the *Marmasastra*, is also incorporated in performance in many ways; as a result, most of the performance forms in Kerala show a meticulous knowledge of the human body in terms of anatomy, movements and also the ways in which the body is prepared and nourished through systematic approaches. The physical training methods are equally informed by these native medical systems as are the performances themselves. One aspect of training is regular oil massage as prescribed in *Ayurveda*. The oil is prepared using a selection of herbs combined depending on the physical nature of the actor's body.

As far as breathing techniques are concerned, they are vital to acting and therefore central to actor training. In *Kudiyattam*, for example, the expression of the nine *rasas* is each associated with a specific breathing pattern. *Kudiyattam* is the performance form that I am going to look at in the following sections because breath in terms of training and performance are much more evident in *Kudiyattam* than in any other performance forms in Kerala.

3.1.1 Breath and the *Natyasastra*

Bharata incorporates almost all the systems of knowledge, including *Ayurveda* and *Vastu*, architecture, available at his time in the *Natyasastra* at various points to enhance and elaborate the theory and practice of theatre. The medical knowledge of *Ayurveda* is incorporated in the physical training section of the *Natyasastra* suggesting various herbal medicines to prepare the oil for massaging the actors. *Kāmasūtra*, the knowledge of sex, has been brought into discussion when Bharata explains the types of heroines as to how they appear and what their emotional temperaments and characteristic behavioural features are. Similarly, the second chapter of the *Natyasastra* elaborately discusses architectural principles in the context of building playhouses of different sizes and shapes. In chapters eleven, twelve and thirteen, Bharata explains various styles and patterns of postures which clearly take their origin in *Yoga*. The *Natyasastra* thus offers an interdisciplinary methodology to understand, analyse and practice theatre.

In this interdisciplinary context, breath is mentioned in the *Natyasastra* in Chapter eight when Bharata discusses various nostril movements in relation to facial acting, the acting of emotions. He explains six types of nostril movements as *nata, manta, vikrista, sochwasa, vikunita* and *swabhaviki*. Shrinking the nose is *nata*, stability without movement is *manta*, expansion is *vikrista*, inhalation is *sochwasa*, distortion is *vikunita*, and the normal state is *swabhaviki*. Bharata provides examples of how each nostril mode or movement is to be used in acting emotions: actors are to show *nata* (shrinking of the nose) when they need to show crying silently, or being deep in thoughts and in a sorrowful state of mind. The experience of strong unpleasant smells, anger and fear will be shown by *vikrista* (expansion), whereas pleasant smells and all the emotions expressed through sigh will be followed by *sochwasa* (inhalation). When actors need to show jealousy they will use *vikunita* (distorted). All other emotions are supported by *swabhaviki* (the normal state) (NS. 8: 123-128). Bharata thus establishes the link between nostrils (and indirectly, therefore, breath) and emotions. A further reference to breath in the *Natyasastra* follows in the section on movement training in chapter eleven. Here, Bharata says that the proper habit of eating healthy food and the proper ways of physical training are the basis of strengthening *prana*, the breath, without which the actor's work would not accomplish perfection (*siddhi*) (NS.e 11: 85). There are no further details in the *Natyasastra* exploring the training of breath. These two examples, however, suggest that Bharata was aware of the importance of breath in acting.

Bharata's incorporation of *yogic* methodology and breath in the *Natyasastra* can be understood further by looking at the definitions of *rasa*, and *Yoga* in relation to the *rasa sutra* in the *Natyasastra*, the verse explaining the meaning of *rasa: Vibhava- anubhava-vyabhicaribhava-samyogad rasa-nispattih. Rasa* emerges through the union (samyogad) of the three elements that constitute theatre: specific situations in the play (*vibhava*), expressed by the actor's body (*anubhava*) and the actor's mental states (*vyabhicaribhava*). Meyer-Dinkgräfe's reassessment of these terms leads to the conclusion that the aim of both *Yoga* and *rasa* is to access the inaccessible and an extended level of extra-daily experience through working with physical and mental properties involved in daily life. Breath has been identified as an element of transformation in both practices (*Yoga*, see Chapter two and *rasa* according to the *Natyasastra*).

3.1.2 Breath and *Rasa*

The *Natyasastra* establishes the links between breath and acting to achieve the experience of *rasa* in the audience theoretically. *Kudiyattam* offers practical methods of training breath. *Kudiyattam* is the only surviving Sanskrit theatre tradition restored in the temple theatres of Kerala, and so far there are no studies adequately showing what elements *Kudiyattam* carries forward from Sanskrit tradition and what elements have been incorporated from local traditions. Perhaps it might be both and therefore, it is difficult to isolate the original source of the breath-related practice found in *Kudiyattam*. Studying these practices of breath in *Kudiyattam* allows us to draw parallels between meditation techniques and acting techniques that are integrated into the performance structure of *Kudiyattam*.

The style of acting in *Kudiyattam* is very much dependent on the expressivity of the actor's eyes and the twenty-one movement patterns of the eyes. Breath in turn is central to eye training. As Mani Madhava Chakyar, the legendary master performer explains, eye training is carried out by sitting crossed-legged, applying *ghee* to the eyelids, massaging the eyes by stretching them sideways and pushing the upper eyelids as much as possible with the fingers.[7] Chakyar explains the role of breath in eye training as follows:

> When the student gets rather well trained in these movements, the rest of the eye training involving breath (*vayu*) in the pupil of the eyes depends entirely on the skill and practice of the teacher. While doing this complicated 'vayu exercises' special care should be taken to avoid squint-eye. The training should make the student bring 3 vayus in his [her] eyes. Only after the completion of this training does the actor become capable of expressing adequate *rasa* in his [her] acting.[8]

Here, Chakyar describes a specific technique of applying breath to the eyes. The training of *Kudiyattam* will be completed only after the successful learning of this specific technique of bringing the breath to the eyes. According to Chakyar, the *rasa* can only be expressed adequately by bringing breath to the eyes, which means that breath is a vital element in rasa acting.[9] Another master teacher of *Kudiyattam*, P.K.Narayanan Nambiar confirms these observations by adding that the subtle and complex acting techniques in *Kudiyattam* very much rely upon breath because unless the actor applies *vayu* in the eyes when the mountain Himalaya is shown, the actor's mere imagination of the mountain would leave it devoid of any 'greatness'.[10] The word 'greatness' here suggests the convincing projection of the imaginary objects; the size of an ordinary mountain and the size of Himalaya are different and according to Nambiar, this difference could only be shown through the application of the appropriate amount of *vayu*, breath. The movement patterns of the eyes and other physical movements might be the same in an ordinary mountain and the Himalaya but the breath applied to each situation will be substantially different. This is a very subtle element in the acting of *Kudiyattam* and according to my observations the actor creates various spatial distinctions, through the twenty-one patterns of eye movements such as horizontal, vertical and diagonal while showing the mountain. Following the eye movements in this acting, we sometimes feel the length and shortness of time as well as the depth and heights of the space throughout in the performance, wherever it is necessary, according to the narrative of the mountain Himalaya. The audience can clearly distinguish when the actor looks at the void in the sky and the solid surface in the earth and as the practice is understood at present, the application of breath to the eyes is the key technique involved in this acting.

Usha Nangyar of Iringalakkuda, an actress of the Ammannur School demonstrated and explained the use of breath in *rasa* acting.[11] For her, the approach to breath in *Kudiyattam* acting is neither systematically classified nor theorised in accordance with the traditional scholarship as well as practice. Thus, there is nothing written on it; rather, knowledge is handed down from generation to generation through gurus or heads of schools in each respective style. There is no system of teaching only nine *rasas* separately because traditionally *rasa* acting is taught along with the text while blocking the scenes and therefore, it is obvious that the application of breath in each *rasa* is also taught by the guru as and when it appears in the play. According to Usha the guru will instruct the disciple as to how to breathe and where the breath has to be taken in showing some particular *rasa* and then it is the duty of the pupil to nourish it through 128 own effort and hard work. I record the application of breath in each *rasa* as suggested by Usha Nangyar as follows:

1. *Erotic*: Taking breath down from the lower abdomen and pushing it slowly and gradually up until it reaches at the middle centre of the head.

2. *Marvellous*: Taking breath down from the lower abdomen and pushing it rapidly and constantly up until it flows through the nostrils. Holding the breath, after a while, with no movements can also be part of expressing this *rasa*.

3. *Comic:* Taking it from the lower abdomen and bringing it to the middle of the chest and shaking it while the outer flow breaks constantly.

4. *Pathetic:* Taking it from the lower tip of the vertebral column (*muladhara*) and pushing it up slowly until it reaches the middle of the chest and then compressing it without an up-and-down movement. When this breath is taken from the bottom make sure that you feel a slight sensation at the bottom tip and the same with the neck when you compress it in the chest. These sensations indicate the proper directions of breath.

5. *Furious:* Taking the breath from the lower abdomen and bringing it up until it reaches the neck, then compressing it vigorously in the throat, and exhaling through eyes. An exercise is suggested to achieve this breathing pattern, which consists in compressing breath in the throat and exhaling through the eyes.

6. *Heroic:* Taking breath exactly from the back of the belly button, pushing it strongly up forward until it reaches the top back of the shoulder bones and then holding it firmly and compressing it all over the back side.

7. *Odious:* Taking it from the lower abdomen and pushing it through both nostrils strongly and rapidly. Two exercises are suggested to achieve this pattern: 1. shrinking the whole face while pushing the entire breath out from inside, which is the pattern of breathing in this *rasa* 2. Expanding the whole face

while inhaling slowly and gently, which is the pattern of breathing for the odious *rasa*.

8. *Terrible:* Taking breath from the lower tip of the vertebral column, pushing it firmly and strongly up until it reaches the throat area and then compressing it down.

9. *Santa*[12]*:* Taking breath from the lower tip of the vertebral column and slowly pushing it up until it reaches the crown of the head while withdrawing your eyes from the sight and ears from hearing. An exercise is suggested to achieve this pattern of breathing, which is looking at a closer distance and then at a longer distance while pushing the eyes out and pulling them in with the help of breath.

The breathing patterns described for each *rasa* are different from one another and each one operates by using specific body regions. We can see a general pattern emerging out of this practice: breath is taken mostly either from the lower abdomen or from the lower tip of the vertebral column, and then arrested, compressed and released through different body regions depending on the nature of the *rasa*. Nangyar adds that breath does not have an independent status in acting: rather it always goes alongside emotions. In other words, breath naturally moves along with emotions and knowing the basic source and movements of breathing will give the performer perfect control over the emotions: specific emotions can be highlighted through controlling and redirecting breath. This process requires hard working and long-term creative involvement. Regarding the movement of breath in each *rasa*, Nangyar uses *yogic* metaphors to explain the movement of breath starting from the lower tip of the vertebral column and terminating in the crown of the head. While Nangyar provides such detailed descriptions of the links between emotions and breathing, which she learnt from her guru, she does not know anything about the origins or development of this technique. I will address the missing link, the relation between performance and meditation techniques, particularly, *yogic* methods, in Chapter four.

3.1.3 *Svara-Vayu*: A Lost Tradition of Breath

Usha Nangyar learned the technique of *Svara-vayu* from Guru Ammannur Madhava Chakyar, the master performer not only of the Iringalakkuda style but of the whole of *Kudiyattam*. Chakyar underwent training with Guru Kunjunny Tampuran, the King of Kodungalloor.[13] Tampuran was well versed in Sanskrit, as well as *Ayurveda*, *Yoga*, *Jyothish* (astrology), music and the *Natyasastra*. Ammannur explains the training of breath that he underwent with Tampuran:

> My training under him usually began at 3.p.m. Focussing the eyes on a near object and then on a distant object and the eye exercises (*netrabhinaya*) related to them was the first lesson. Then came the expression of the nine *rasa*s. The basic emotions (*sthayibhava)* corresponding to each *rasa* had to be clearly grasped first. The breathing has to be regulated in a special way to produce each of these *rasa*s on the face. The *rasa-bhava* becomes clearer and more expressive when it is accompanied by the right method of breath control. This was Tampuran's style of acting emptions. In *rasabhinaya*, the actor must know when to accentuate the *rasa* and when to mitigate it to suit the context. This requires long and steady practice of the method called *svara-vayu.*[14]

Ammannur confirms the existence of a breath-related training method in the acting of *rasa* in *Kudiyattam* through a method known as *svara-vayu.*[15] The word *svara* means the resonant voice in music and *vayu* means breath; therefore, *svara-vayu* is a method in which the basics of music is brought into acting through breath or breathing in accordance with the notes of music. This method goes back to the *Natyasastra* where Bharata explains seven basic musical notes in relation to *rasa* in Chapter nineteen while elaborating the delivery of lines in a play. Bharata lists the seven *svaras* as follows*: shadja, rishabha, gandhara, madhyama, panchama, dhaivata* and *nishada* (NS. 19: 40). The *Natyasastra* further emphasises the application of these *svaras* in accordance with the appropriate production and distribution of *rasa*, and Bharata offers some examples showing which *svara* is adequate in producing which *rasa*:

1. *Hasya* and *Shringara*: *madhyama* and *panchama*

2. *Veeram*, *raudram* and *atbhutam*: *shadja* and *rishabha*

3. *Karuman*: *gandhara* and *nishada*
4. *Bibhalsa* and *bhayanaka*: *dhaivata* (NS. 19: 40)

Bharata does not elaborate further about how each *svara* is connected to each *rasa* and how to explore this connection between music and *rasa*. However, eminent *Kathakali* performer Tekkinkattil Ramunni Nair, dedicated a whole chapter in his 1955 book *Natyarcana* to expaining the methodology.[16] While interpreting Bharata's views on *rasa* and *svara*, Nair explains the *svara-vayu* technique. *Bhava* is the un-manifest base of *rasa* and only the proper application of *svara-vayu* brings the accurate expression of *rasa*: without this application of *vayu*, *bhava* would not turn into *rasa*, and the actor would not seem present on the stage. *Vayu*, in this sense, is the basis of manifested *rasa* mediating between basic *bhava* and the expressed *rasa*. The application of s*vara- vayu* can be divided into two stages:

1. Application of breath along with spoken words, which is the stylised rendering of Sanskrit verses, composed according to the musical notes mentioned above, in the case of classical performance like *Kudiyattam*. Here, the application of each *svara* to its appropriate *rasa*, as suggested by Bharata, is more direct and simple.

2. Application of breath to the eyes to produce *rasa* in a dramatic situation through silent moments without words.

S*vara-vayu* is said to be the life force of *rasa* acting, which is practiced in *Kudiyattam* and *Kathakali*, the performance traditions of Kerala and the King of Kodungalloor is supposed to be the originator of this technique. What is the practice of *svara-vayu* and how can a particular pattern of breathing be associated with the expression of a particular *rasa*? T. K. Rammunni Nair explains the practical methodology on three levels: according to the *svara-vayu* system, the actor has to understand the following aspects before applying breath to acting:

Stage I

1. The details of the basic emotion *(bhava)* of the character in general as well as in the context of particular situations in the play.

2. The actions and reactions through gestures and movements planned for the character (*anubhava*).

3. The eye movements in relation to the proposed *rasa* (which is more important in classical forms like *Kudiyattam* because *rasa* is enacted predominantly through eyes).

4. All the subtle transitory mental states of the character running along with basic emotions and their actions and reactions.

Stage II

Then the actor should carefully choose adequate *svaras* appropriate for the *rasa*s intending to show the character she is playing. This applies to both verbal and non-verbal acting and the actor should identify *svaras* in connection with *rasas* considering the character, situations, play, and all the details of the actions, reactions and the transitory mental states.

Stage III

The third stage will be identifying specific breathing patterns associated with the selected *svaras*. Once the breathing pattern is identified, the actor should reproduce these physical patterns consciously in acting, specifically with thoughts, emotional changes and physical movements in acting. This approach brings the expression of proper *rasa*. This is the way *svara-vayu* is explained in relation to *rasa* acting in *Kudiyattam*. No *Kudiyattam* scholar in Kerala knows whether it is a Sanskrit tradition or an aspect of local knowledge incorporated in the performance later on. Perhaps that historical question is irrelevant in this context because the technique that is mentioned in the *Natyasastra* can be found as a living performance tradition in Kerala. In my acquaintance and knowledge of academic and performance practice, I have never come across such a practical interpretation of the *Natyasastra* shedding new light on *rasa* and *breath*. This is one example of how Keralan performance tradition is significant because the rich repertoire of performance forms and the Sanskrit scholarship brought by the *Namboothiris* (Brahmins) have integrated in a more highly sophisticated and imaginative manner than in any other regions of India. Therefore, the performance tradition as well as the knowledge system related to it is developed intricately by incorporating several other systems available in both regional languages and Sanskrit. This historical significance of Keralan performance tradition is suggested by Abhinavagupta. In his *Abhinavabharathi* he suggests that his *rasa* interpretation of the *Natyasastra* was written down in response to questions raised by actors from Kerala. In addition, the palm leaf manuscripts of the entire plays of Bhasa, the most renowned of the Sanskrit playwrights, have been discovered in Kerala; *Kudiyattam*, the oldest existing theatre form in the world has been performed continuously in the theatres built inside temples throughout Kerala. *Svara-vayu* has to be added to this list as a unique method developed in Kerala by incorporating elements of the *Natyasastra, Yoga, Kudiyattam* and music.

Although *svara-vayu* is explained by T.K Ramunni Nair, the only person who has direct contact to this method is Ammannur, the legendary performer of *Kudiyattam*. His performances obviously give proof to the application of breath. I asked him about *svara-vayu* in a personal interview (July 2003). He responded that music was the key methodological base for the King of Kodungalloor to develop *svara-vayu* but "I was not a musician, he did not teach me this method", and then he explained a slightly different approach to *svara-vayu:*

> When a man dies a natural death, that death is preceded by the operation of the three *vayus* (climacteric breathing), *chinnan, mahan* and *urdhan*. If an actor can operate these three *vayus* accurately in their proper order and strength he can enact death very well. He taught me this method of imitating death. As a result of learning this *abhinaya*, I was able to elaborate in the acting of death when I was playing the role of Bali (the monkey King in *Ramayana*) in *Balivadham Kudiyattam.*[17]

This account clearly shows the integration of *Yoga* and *Ayurveda* in *rasa* acting because the types of human breathing, like *chinnan, mahan* and *urdhan* are systematically categorized and explained in these systems of knowledge. As Ammannur also said, he observed closely the death of his mother, giving particular attention to her final breathing to study this further in a real situation. Only on the basis of this experience was he confident in using the method learned from the King of Kodungalloor because he could see that this method was based in real life. It is a very interesting and important observation firstly because the actor of a highly stylised theatrical form like *Kudiyattam* seems to be using a very naturalistic methodological approach to acting which we might expect from Stanislavski. Secondly, what Ammannur further contributes to this knowledge system is to add a practical base to T. K. Ramunni Nair's theoretical explanation of the methodology of *svara-vayu*. However, Ammannur does not seem to know the *svara-vayu* system as it is explained by T. K. Ramunni Nair because of his lack of knowledge in music. Thus we can conclude that there was a system in Kerala practiced by the actors in the classical forms of theatre like *Kudiyattam* and *Kathakali.* The knowledge of this system did not transfer properly to the next generation of actors. What Ammannur knows is not the *svara-vayu*, as he said, but something he developed on his own particularly to perform the death of the Monkey King. Usha Nangyar was trained by Ammannur, but the knowledge is again only partly transferred because the death of the Monkey King is only enacted by male actors and therefore, there is no chance for Nangyar to learn that technique.

I still remember watching Ammannur performing the death of the monkey King sixteen years back in a traditional playhouse (*Kuthambalam*) in Trichur when I was an undergraduate student of theatre. I never knew that death can be performed for so long and with such incredible detail. He created a particular audible rhythm through his breathing along with his acting that mesmerised the audience for not less than one and half to two hours. This might be one of the wonders in the world of acting that an actor can hold the attention of the audience for hours by sitting and acting death. It is unfortunate, then, that no one has been trained by him to perform this character as he does and this knowledge will vanish forever when this 85-year-old actor is no more. The point that I am trying to make here is that what we know at present in *Kudiyattam* under the name of *svara-vayu* is a limited understanding of a larger knowledge developed by a dedicated researcher, the King of Kodungalloor, by using several systems of knowledge and practice like medicine, music and spirituality along with the *Natyasastra*. Neither of Ammannur's disciples nor the Guru himself seems to understand *svara-vayu* in its full depth as it is described by T. K. Ramunni Nair. As G. Venu, the *Kathakali* performer and the researcher of *Kudiyattam*, puts it:

> Tampuran could not find in any of his disciples the desired combination of musician and actor...that must be the reason why he did not pass on the *svara-vayu* technique to any one.[18]

So, in the final analysis, the following conclusions can be drawn:

1. Breath is mentioned in the *Natyasastra* in several occasions but it is explained mostly in relation to music and *rasa*. But the practice of this is unknown.

2. A practical approach based on Bharata called *svara-vayu* has been developed by Kunjunni Tampuran, the King of Kodungalloor and practiced by the actors of *Kudiyattam* and *Kathakali*. The method seems to be interdisciplinary as it incorporates knowledge from medicine, meditation and music.

3. The system has not been transferred accurately to the next generation of actors but it is partly understood by Ammannur Madhava Chakyar of Iringalakkuda who learned some breathing techniques from the King of Kodungalloor but not *svara-vayu* because of the lack of his knowledge in music.

The *svara-vayu* method is lost forever. The key associations established in this method between performance and *yogic* practice and between breath and *rasa* acting are vital to my thesis. Therefore I wish to relate an incident which might suggest some deeper influence that a *Siddha Yogi* made in the life and thoughts of Kunjunni Tampuran, the King of Kodungalloor. The most important contribution of Tampuran to acting in *Kudiyattam* was his deep exploration of *santa rasa*, proposing that all other *rasa*s emerge and submerge in *santa* because it is neutral (See Chapter four). Guru Ammannur recalls the story of a *Siddha Yogi* that Tampuran used to tell his disciples. Tampuran happened to meet the *Yogi*, sitting in profound meditation and Tampuran had said that he had seen the perfection of *santa rasa* on that ascetic's serene countenance.[19] Tampuran himself was said to be a *Yogi* and had profound knowledge in the practice of *Yoga*: so the *Siddha Yogi* and some unknown practice of breathing might have inspired the King of Kodungalloor to devise *svara-vayu* to establish the practical links between *santa rasa* and *yogic* meditation.

A contemporary observation serves as confirmation of this assumption: in Usha Nangyar's demonstration of *santa rasa* I noticed that she does not breathe during her acting. She does not recognise that she is not breathing, and she does not feel any discomfort because of it. Her breathless state during her acting of *santa rasa* seems to be similar to *Siddha Yoga* breathing called *Restoration of Breath,* which I am going to discuss in the following chapter. Finally, *Kudiyattam* exemplifies evidence that a systematic practice of breath in acting existed in the classical performance traditions in Kerala, informed by Bharata as well as *Siddha Yoga* of South India, but the tradition is irrecoverably lost.

3.1.4. *Noh* in Contemporary Actor Training

In Japanese culture, the traditional knowledge of breathing has been employed to train actors. Yoshi Oida suggests techniques derived from *Noh* training:[20]

1. Stand or sit comfortably with your back straight, breathe in slowly through the nose, breathe out through the mouth, but as you breathe out imagine that the air passes out through the pores of the skin.

2. To develop this further, imagine that the air enters the body through the navel and exits through the pores.

3. Concentrate your breathing in the *hara,* the area just below your navel, and imagine that the air is entering your body through the feet, then it travels to the *hara*. Exhale, and visualise the breath leaving the body through the *tan-den,* the core point of the *hara*, about three centimetres below the navel.

4. When you breathe in, imagine that you are saying 'aaaah' and that when you breathe out you use the sound 'aawm' (or 'ohm'). You can reverse the sounds, 'aaaah' on the out-breath, and 'aawm' as you inhale.

5. Use a real voiced sound on the out-breath, using these various combinations. For example, breathe in with imaginary 'aawm' through the navel, and out with the real sound 'aaah' through the navel.

6. Breathe in through the left nostril and out through the right. Then reverse the process. This can be done by pressing your finger against the opposite nostril in order to hold it shut.

Oida suggests more breathing exercises that are derived from *Noh* drama and *T'ai Ch'i* in which breathing is explored through imagination, use of the voiced sounds and specific bodily zones. He used these techniques to train the actors in Brook's production of *The Mahabharata*. In my analysis, the use of left and right nostril breathing, the voiced sound, the exploration of bodily zones like the navel region all are similar to the practice proposed by *Yoga*. In his book, *The Invisible Actor,* Oida has included these breathing techniques in the section of speaking by giving much emphasis on voice training. The knowledge of the East on breath, and Eastern breathing practice, found in several forms of spiritual and physical traditions such as meditation, martial arts, and performance have served as sources of reference and inspiration for contemporary Western actor training.

3.2 Breath in Western Actor Training

The investigation of the integration of breath in the Western training is largely based on 20th century actor training including some recent trends developed in the 21st century. This is mainly because of two reasons: the ancient methods of training are not fully known and actor training as a systematic discipline developed in Europe and America in the 20th century.

3.2.1 Jacques Copeau (1879-1949)

Jacques Copeau works between breath and text using 'voluntary control' over an 'involuntary' nature of human breathing. Breathing, for Copeau, "is an involuntary, essentially natural, life-sustaining activity,"[21] which he called *primum mobile*; it is the basis of gestural sincerity and vocal concord. Breath controls everything and "a voice which does not breathe becomes dull, collapses on itself and becomes sad". It is dragged along by the text, which ensures that "our sensibility has the faculty to move in any direction". In the context of the actor's presence Copeau says that "inadequate breathing creates disorders... [and] vigorous breathing brings freedom". His practical examples in relation to breathing are related to exploring the text through "tonality, postures and rhythm". Breath controls everything, for Copeau, and his approach tends towards identifying techniques of using breath in delivering the text successfully and convincingly. As Copeau explains this, "reading out loud requires perpetual *tours de force* of breathing… [particularly], when a dramatic text demands constant switching from one tone to another, from one movement to another" In his system Copeau intends to develop a method of reading the text by exploring actor's physicality, the dynamics of the changing attitudes of the range of tonality, posture and rhythm involved in the text. Copeau's ultimate intention was not just to create physical fitness in the actor's body but a physical training that would be integral to the development of the actor as an instrument. When he says that the actors should not 'get wrapped up' in the text, what he meant was a physical culture helping the actors to unlock the text visually and audibly. Copeau explained *neutrality* as "a point of departure of an expression" a "state of repose, of calm of relaxation or decontraction, of silence or simplicity." Copeau does not establish any link between breath and the actor's neutral state of mind. As John Rudlin observes, in today's world, we are more informed by disciplines like *Yoga* and *T'ai Ch'i* about how breath works in neutrality and relaxation by exploring the dynamics between breathing and movement: Copeau's understanding of actor's breathing, therefore, is elementary.[22]

3.2.2 Stanislavski: Breath and Sub-text

Stanislavski refers to the actor's breathing when he explained the concept of *sub-text* hidden beneath the words. The term describes anything that the character feels or thinks or does, which cannot be put into words. According to Stanislavski, actors communicate subtext through the non-verbal communication of their body language, intonations and pauses. As Sharon Marie Carnicke argues, Stanislavski, under the influence of *Yoga*, thought about the actors' non-verbal communication as the transmitting and receiving of *rays of energy*, which are like "psychic radio waves."[23] Stanislavski believed that in every exhalation we send rays out into the environment and with every inhalation we receive energy back into our bodies. Non-verbal communication, for Stanislavski, is the firm grounding for the actor's use of words as the element of communication. He believed that non-verbal expression can be controlled through systematic application of the rays of energy. He taught actors the ways to recognise and manipulate the rays of energy in order to enhance their non-verbal communication. The following are the exercises suggested by Stanislavski (p.22):

1. Close your eyes, relax, and feel your breath moving through your body. Visualise the breath as warm, yellow sunlight, energising you. As you inhale, the light is travelling from the top of your head down to your toes; as you exhale, reverse the direction of the breath.

2. Close your eyes, relax, and feel your breath moving through your body. As you inhale, breathe the energy in from the surrounding room; as you exhale, send the energy back out into the furthest corner.

3. Stand apart from the group, hands held with palms outward. Radiate energy from your hands to someone else in the room. Does anyone in the room feel a transmission?

4. Actors stand in a single file, one behind the other. The person behind concentrates on a simple command (open the door, sit down, shake my hand), then radiates it to the person in front, who carries out the command.

Stanislavski works with silent moments and non-verbal communication in order to link actors' breathing into theatrical communication, an approach which is crucial to enhance the actor's expressive quality rooted in her body-mind dynamics. Another significance of Stanislavski's understanding of the role of breathing in actor training is that he establishes a link between the flow of breath and the flow of energy into the theatrical communication through the actor's non-verbal physical work. *Yoga* forms the basis of Stanislavski's breath-related exercises and an analysis of those exercises leads to the following conclusions:

1. Sub-text is conveyed through actor's physicality by means of non-verbal communication.

2. Breathing as the source of energy creates psychic radio waves in the body, called rays of energy, which enable the actor to communicate beyond the conventional modes of theatrical expression, beyond the body. Stanislavski wanted to work with actor on their psychic levels, aiming to enable them to influence their fellow-actors on stage.

Rays of energy created through breathing link the psycho-physical elements in the body and then move further onto a higher level of communication between the actors, within a theatrical context, focusing more on the psychic impulses than the physical body.

3.2.3 Grotowski and Breath

Grotowski refers to breath on several occasions, mainly in relation to voice training, and at times in connection with Artaud. He does not mention Stanislavski in terms of breath. Influenced by *Yoga*, Grotowski believed that abdominal diaphragmatic breathing is the perfect type of human respiration because this is the fundamental type of breathing found with children, animals and people who are closer to nature.[24] There is no single authentic type of breathing suitable for everyone, nor for all physical and psychic situations. As he puts it:

> Breathing is a physiological reaction linked with specific characteristics in each of us and which is dependent on situations, type of effort, physical activities. It is the natural thing for most people, when breathing freely, to use abdominal respiration. The number of types of abdominal respiration, however, are unlimited…If the actor tries artificially to impose on himself the perfect, objective abdominal respiration, he blocks the natural process of respiration, even if his is naturally of the diaphragmatic type.[25]

On another occasion he suggests that if the actor has enough air to speak and sing, "why then create a problem by imposing on him a different type of respiration?"[26]

Let us look at two examples quoted from Grotowski's breathing exercises, from his actor training (1959-1962) section in *Towards a Poor Theatre*.[27]

1. "Method adopted from Hatha Yoga. The vertebral column must be quite straight and for this it is necessary to lie on a hard surface. Block one nostril with a finger and breathe in through the other. When breathing out do the contrary: blocked the nostril through which you breathed in before and breathe out through the one which was blocked at the beginning. The three phases succeed one another in the following rhythm:

    - Inspiration: 4 seconds
    - Hold the breath 12 seconds
    - Expiration 8 seconds"

2. "The method which follows, taken from Classical Chinese theatre, is basically the most effective and can be used in any position where as the previous one necessitates lying down.[28] While standing, place the hands on the two lowest ribs. Inspiration must give an impression of beginning in the very spot where the hands are placed (therefore pushing them outwards) and, continuing through the thorax, produce a sensation that the air column reaches right up to the head. (This means that when breathing in the abdomen and lower ribs dilate first, followed, in smooth succession by the chest). The abdominal wall is then contracted while the ribs remain expanded, thus forming a base for the air stored up and preventing it from escaping with the first words uttered. The abdominal wall (contracting inwards) pulls in the opposite direction to the muscles which expand the lower ribs (contracting outwards), keeping them thus for as long as possible during expiration. Expiration takes place inversely: from the head, through the thorax, to the spot where the palms of the hands are placed. Care must be taken not to compress the indrawn air too much and –as already mentioned- the whole process must take place smoothly…An exercise such as this is not intended to teach respiration for respiration's sake, but prepares for a respiration that will "carry" the voice. It also teaches how to establish a base (the abdominal wall) which, by contracting, allows the easy and vigorous emission of the air and thus the voice."

Grotowski proposes that these breathing exercises help the actor improve their voice power; therefore, at least two of the key elements are missing in Grotowski's understanding of the use of breath in actor training:

1. Regarding the implications of breath in actor training, Stanislavski and Artaud went beyond the level of voice training, arguing that breath enhances subtle physical and psychic expressions as well as a different level of energy and individual consciousness in the actor. Stanislavski believed that breath is the rays of energy through which the actor

enacts the subtext. Artaud's comments on breathing suggest an extended level of extra-daily consciousness, which the actor can experience by employing specific breathing patterns. In both views, breath is understood as the basic source of actor's energy that has direct implications for non-verbal emotional acting. Grotowski does not seem to be taking any insights from these views.

2. Though Grotowski adopted breathing techniques from classical Indian and Chinese traditions, he paid no attention to either the traditional Eastern philosophy of breathing or its the proper practice

These examples suggest that Grotowski was little concerned with breath and unaware of the importance and dynamics of breath in the actor's body-mind. Grotowski considered the actor's body as a medium that needs to be trained properly to break the usual habits of using the body so as to enable it to represent deeper impulses of psychic life. However, he never fully considered breath as something which could be trained in order to help the actors either to achieve a different level of understanding the function of the body and mind or to feel them experiencing the emergence of a different level of energy explored through breathing.

3.2.4 Jacques Lecoq

Jacques Lecoq identified *equilibrium and respiration* as the extreme limits of all movements applicable to the actor's performance. In the context of movement techniques, Lecoq illustrated examples of the application of breath in the actor's varying attitudes:[29]

1. The farewell: in a standing position, I raise my arm to the vertical to wave goodbye to someone.

2. If this movement is made while breathing in as the arm is raised, and then breathing out as it falls back, the sense of a positive farewell result.

3. If you do the opposite, raising the arm on the out breath, and letting it fall as you breathe in, the dramatic state becomes a negative: I do not want to say goodbye, but I am obliged to do so.

4. Another possibility: breathe in, hold your breath, then do the movement, and only breathe out once it is completed, which gives rise to an emotionless salute.

5. Finally the opposite is also possible: breathe out, then do the movement, and only breath in once it is completed, which also gives rise to an emotion less state.

As Lecoq explains, this is one example of the nuances of breath control applied to the nine attitudes; breath control has a profound effect on the dramatic justifications, which are left with the students to discover further for themselves. Lecoq's observations on breath are very important when we look at how breath works, deeply interweaving with the actor's bodily movements and emotional attitudes. Lecoq's methods evokes some distant associations to at least two systems: *rasa* acting in *Kudiyattam* where nine emotions are acted with the help of several patterns of controlling breath and some ancient meditation techniques reinvented by Osho showing how daily mental attitudes and activities are closely connected to the incoming and outgoing breaths and how those emotional attitudes can be altered and changed by bringing control over daily respiration. I will discuss this meditation technique in the following section to clarify John Martin's observations about breath—Martin explains the links between breath, physical actions and emotional attitudes with reference to Lecoq's techniques.

3.2.5 Recent Views

The role of breath in training and performance has been discussed by a number of practitioners and academics in more recent times. John Martin, in *The Intercultural Performance Handbook*[30] explains some of the breathing exercises he developed during his long years of intercultural practice of training and performance. The most focused areas of his training method are: centre of the body, breathing and eye movements. Martin defines four basic states of breathing: *Breathing in, breathing out, breathing held in* and *breathing held out*. Breathing in or out are active breathing and breathing held in or out are passive breathing. He further establishes the link between the energy level of the body and breath: the weakest energy level is when breath is passive, held out, the energy level is weak during active breathing in, there is limited strength when the breath is passive, held in and the highest level of energy is achieved during active breathing out. Martin explains that "the active breathing-out allows you to repeat an action time and time again."[31] Laborious work like loading sacks and wielding a sledge-hammer would need this kind breathing. He further relates these four ways of breathing to gestures and emotions:

1. Breathing in for welcoming and seeing someone arriving.

2. Breathing out for saying goodbye and sadness.

3. Held-in breath for expressing surprise and shock

4. Held-out breath to express powerlessness and depression.

These exercises are similar to Lecoq's nine attitudes. Lecoq suggests four combinations of breathing in relation to *farewell*, an exercise establishing the links between breathing and emotions, which has enormous impact on Martin's breath work.

Martin, then, provides several exercises exploring breath in terms of the actor's body and emotion such as "states and energies within breathing" and "breathing and gestures"; his understanding of breath is physical and he attempts to bring in generalisations about breath based on his intercultural observations. He does not, however, provide explanations for those observed states or modes of breath. According to the South Indian *Siddha* tradition, breath is deeper than physiology; it is the pure substance of our being. As a *Siddha* Yogi once explained a subtle aspect of breathing to me,[32] breath usually goes in and out naturally and there is a subtle gap in between the two: this gap is said to be the centre because it is neutral, neither active nor passive—potential and neutral. One gap occurs after the breath has come in and before it goes out again, and another gap after the breath has gone out and before it comes in again. The *Siddha* tradition proposes several ways in which one can utilise the existence of the gap: opening it up to direct experience leads to a considerable increase of energy. Similarly, Chinese martial artists are trained to be always in that gap to enhance their performance through exploring the vital neutral energy. This is why complete breathing out gives an extraordinary sense of strength. Yogis said to be in that state of complete neutrality are always without any action, mental or physical. In Chapter four I will discuss this further in terms of presence and the pre-expressive.

Martin's observations about breath's physical and emotional implications in the body and mind prove to be appropriate in terms of practice, arrived at by observation and a certain amount of trial and error, but what is obviously missing is a knowledge system which can explain the dynamics of breath involved in the psycho-physicality of the actor. As I observed, this is what is lacking from the contemporary Western understanding of breath: a philosophy and a practice to explain the functioning of breath. Eastern training methods are firmly grounded in this knowledge of breath developed through interdisciplinary interactions between medicine, meditation, martial arts and performance. Martin's training method appears to be one of the best examples of a contemporary intercultural training and theatre practice, from a Western perspective, because this method actively engages theatrical traditions in Asia and Africa in order to create a highly imaginative and spontaneous workshop model.

Phillip Zarrilli's training of *Kalarippayattu* and Nicolas Núñez's *Anthropocosmic Theatre* are the two other recent trends that have to be mentioned here in terms of the practical research they have been doing on breath. According to Zarrilli, the practice of *Kalarippayattu* enables him to enter into a state of heightened awareness by coordinating his body-mind and breath through the highly codified movements of the Keralan martial arts form.[33] While comparing *Kalarippayattu* with another Chinese martial form *T'ai Ch'i*, Zarrilli argues that proper breath control through inhalation and exhalation is almost evident and parallel to the physical movements of the forms and therefore, any physical exploration in these forms naturally explores breath as well. He uses selective breathing exercises from *Yoga* along with martial arts movement techniques to enhance the capacity of controlling breath. What Zarrilli aims to achieve in his research is to establish "the link between breath and the body-in-motion", which he considers the basis of the movement pattern of both *Kalarippayattu* and *T'ai Ch'i.*[34] He also explains how a *Kathakali* performer is able to perform emotional states through facial expressions by manipulating breath along with the movements of the eyebrows and facial muscles.[35] Bringing in Artaud's views of the existence of a breathing pattern parallel to physical and mental movements, Zarrilli argues that breathing in the form of controlling inhalation and exhalation is very much present in the *rasa* acting in *Kathakali*: "throughout this process the breathing is deep and connected through the entire body via the "root of the navel" (*nābhi mūla*), that is, it is not shallow chest breathing."[36] Thus Zarrilli's argument is about a deep abdominal breathing, which runs throughout and controls the actor's physical and emotional levels. I can draw two key propositions from his research:

1. The links between breathing and movements are established in the martial arts like *Kalarippayattu* and *T'ai Ch'i* through controlling breath through inhalation and exhalation.

2. Breathing in the form of controlling inhalation and exhalation is very much present in the *rasa* acting in *Kathakali.*

Zarrilli's understanding of the ways in which breath works in *Kalarippayattu, T'ai Ch'I* and *Kathakali* seems to be accurate in the sense that all these forms, one way or other, integrate breath controlling along side with physical movements and emotional expressions. A deep abdominal breathing is also characteristic to the physical nature of all the forms he mentioned in his research. But, there is a lack of a philosophical system or a concept or a practical method to explain the dynamics of breath involved in the actor's body.

Nicolas Núñez points out that the tools of breathing, movement, participation and vibration are the firm basis of Anthropocosmic theatre. "The deep breathing" and the "unity of consciousness" are the two key elements that his theatre approach is aiming to achieve.[37] He also mentions a certain type of breathing pattern, which is established in his body. Apart from these few references of breathing, he does not offer a training method or a theatre concept based on breath.

In their discussion of the actor's *pre-expressive* level, Malekin and Yarrow reinvestigate the role of breath in training and performance, arguing theoretically that "breath is also a key factor" in understanding the pre-expressive level of actor's consciousness.[38] Breathing exercises derived from Indian and Chinese *yogic* and performance traditions enhance the actor's capacity of breathing, which eventually coordinates rhythm, movement and verse speaking in training and performance:

> "...we are not just talking about control, but about a centring of the breath from the solar plexus area. The crucial factor is the ability to return breath to utter stillness and channel its outflow from there. In passing from the quietest level of breathing to the vital cessation of breath characteristic of *turiya, Samadhi,* etc...[39]

The *yogic* concepts of *turiya* and *samadhi* refer to altered levels of human consciousness and Malekin and Yarrow are linking that extra-daily state into the actor's pre-expressivity, describing that breath is able to "expand the inner space" of the actor, and to create "a specific shift in the physiology, which accompanies a different form of awareness". Although the understanding of the "centred breath" is embedded in a number of performance traditions..."the practice is currently often not fully understood..."[40] While discussing the nature of the ritual act Malekin argues that ritual is not a symbolic action, an externalised signal of an intended meaning, but rather "it is consecration and integration of external action within ultimate unity in keeping with core meaning of 'rite'...and this integration certainly involves the quality of breath..."[41] From a similar point of view, Meyer Dinkgräfe investigates the spiritual links between acting and *yogic* practice, proposing that in order to achieve the quality of *sattva*, the higher level of individual consciousness, the body, mind and spirit have to be united and *Yoga* suggests three approaches to achieve this unity: physical exercises (*asanas)*, breathing exercises (*pranayama)* and meditation.[42] What we see in Malekin, Yarrow and Meyer Dinkgräfe is an important enquiry leading current performance research into new dimensions of the actor's consciousness, exploring hidden depths of the phenomenon of theatrical expression and meaning. As in ritual, if theatre integrates external actions, what kind of stage language would result? (Malekin)? Are there any physiological, psychological and consciousness-related links between an actor, shaman and a *Yogi* (Yarrow)? Is acting a spiritual activity parallel to the *yogic* practice that leads to *yogic* experience (Meyer-Dinkgräfe) What would be the nature of a consciousness-related actor training (Malekin, Yarrow, Meyer Dinkgräfe)? Those are crucial questions they constantly revisit in their writings. All of them have a clear theoretical understanding of the role of breath as a transformational element operates between daily and extra-daily levels of actor's consciousness.

3.2.6 Breath is Meaning: Voice Training

The most popular version of the application of breath in contemporary Western actor training is related to the vocal development of the actor. According to Cicely Berry, "the voice is the means by which you communicate with other people…and it is through the speaking voice that you convey your precise thoughts and feelings."[43] As she further explains, breath is the initial impulse that strikes against the vocal cords in the larynx and makes them vibrate. Sound waves resonate in the chest, the pharynx or hollow space above the larynx in the mouth and nose and bones of the face, and the hollow space in the head, the sinuses. In a chapter called *Relaxation and Breathing,*[44] Berry suggests many exercises helping actors relax the body as well as strengthening the vocal cords to improve the strength and flexibility of the voice. Another aspect of her approach suggests developing the respiratory function by expanding the capacities of the lungs and ribs. Catherine Fitzmaurice's voice work is another notable approach to breath and voice. Susana Bloch's *Alba Emoting* incorporates breathing in terms of providing a physical alternative to emotion. Alba Emoting identifies six basic emotions as the source of all other emotions. The methodological approach to Alba Emoting is based on the three basic aspects of breathing, posture and facial expression.[45] Six basic emotions, joy, anger, sadness, fear, eroticism and tenderness,[46] combine, according to Bloch to numerous further emotions. Each is defined by a specific breathing pattern which she recommends actors to practice to create the corresponding emotion. Bloch's approach establishes links between emotions and specific physical and facial postures. Breath, of course, plays a key role in this psycho-physical approach. However, Alba Emoting as a practical method of training does not explain the functioning of breath in the actor's body and mind as it explains the neuro-physiological level of emotions. Therefore I do not think that a further investigation of these methods, Alba Emoting and voice training, will add anything to the direction of this thesis. The key intention of the thesis is to establish the links between the body, emotions and consciousness of the actor and therefore, the approaches mentioned in this section do not seem helping the development of the basic thoughts and arguments of the thesis.

3.2.7 Exclusion of Breath

Let us also look at few examples of how breath has been excluded by major practitioners. The exclusion of breathing is very much evident in Meyerhold and Joseph Chaikin. For instance, *Shooting from the Bow*, one of the best known exercises in biomechanics is a series of slow moving body stances including a careful use of various body parts like arms, legs and spine followed by sequential pauses. What is not mentioned in this exercise is actor's breathing which runs parallel to all the body movements and pauses mentioned through out in this exercise. Joseph Chaikin's *Sound and Movement Exercise*, as he explains, is a series of movements aiming to "taking a sound and movement out into the space and allowing its form to alter …until the actor recognises or discovers some kind of associative connection with it."[47] There are at least two levels of associative connections at work in this exercise: between the 'inside' and the 'outside' of the actor, and between the body and the mind. According to Dorinda Hulton, what is more important in this is "the flow between the two,"[48] between 'inside' and 'outside' and between the body and mind. But, in this whole exercise, Chaikin refers to breathing only with sound saying that "beginning with the sound of the breath-transforming into a hum- and then into a sung chord in which harmonies and counter-rhythms might develop."[49] Chaikin only considers breathing as the potential source of sound but nothing more than that and not even the flow between 'inside' and 'outside' is mediated by breath. It seems that his approach is more conceptual even working with the body of the actor, which is a characteristic feature running throughout contemporary Western actor training.

Considering other leading figures in 20th century theatre training, Brecht's approach does not seem concerned with the actor's breathing. Peter Brook is predominantly working with well-trained actors from all over the world so, there is no need for Brook developing a training method of his own. Neither Barba nor Richard Schechner seems to have developed any breath-related training. Interestingly, in the entire discussion of 'presence' and 'pre-expressivity', Barba does not mention breath at any stages. This is perhaps the limitation of the anthropological methodology he derived from comparing the physical nature of performance around the world.

In this brief survey of the integration of breath related techniques in the contemporary training and performance the following observations can be charted:

1. Breath is understood in parallel to physical movements. This insight is mainly drawn from *Tai 'Chi* and *Kalarippayattu*.

2. Breath, in particular controlling and arresting of inhalations and exhalations, is used as a tool through which the emotions can be highlighted through. Such practice is inspired by observation of *Yoga*.

3. The existence of some breathing techniques establishing the links between breath and consciousness has been theoretically understood but no proof of practice is available to support the arguments. The theory has not led to the development of practice.

Overall, while some theatre artists have referred to breath and developed some exercises, on the basis of observation and subsequent trial and error, there is no major concept or a method in 20th and 21st century actor training relating to meaningful use of breathing in the context of training the actor's body and mind.

Summary

What we see in Western 20th and 21st century actor training are efforts to understand the dynamics of breath and incorporating them into systems of training. But due to the lack of any in-depth knowledge of the dynamics of breath working in the actor's body, emotion and consciousness, no training method based on breath has been developed systematically. Breath is still understood as an effective tool to train the vocal discipline of the actor. In contrast, traditional Eastern actor training shows evidence of the existence of systematic breath-related training. However, most of those methods have been lost irrecoverably, for example the *svara-vayu* technique. The knowledge of breath-related techniques was kept in the closed circle of family traditions, which made it near impossible for outsiders to gain access to the knowledge and make use of it and record it. In addition, the continuity once safeguarded in the family traditions was broken. In Chapter Four I will explore how breath in its role for performance is related to consciousness. The concept of consciousness will be placed within the context of current debates in consciousness studies. My angle on breath will be mainly with reference to the technique of restoration of breath derived from the *Siddha Yoga* tradition.

Notes

[1] Daniel Meyer-Dinkgräfe, *Approaches to Acting: Past and Present*, London & New York: Continuum, 2001), p. 4.
[2] Ibid., p. 5.
[3] Ibid., p. 7.
[4] Ibid., p. 164.
[5] Suresh Awasthi, *Performance Tradition in India*, (New Delhi: National Book Trust, 2001). p. 64.
[6] Ibid., p. 64.
[7] Mani Madhava Chakyar, "The Training Methods of *Kudiyattam*", in *Sangeet Natak*, (special issue), no. 111-114, p. 49.
[8] Ibid., p. 50.
[9] D. Appukuttan Nair, "*Kudiyattam* and Bhasa" in *Sangeet Natak*, (Special issue), no. 111-114, p. 191.
[10] Interview taken by myself in June 2003.
[11] Interview with the author, June 2003.
[12] Abhinavagupta, the 9th century commentator of the *Natyasastra*, introduced *Santarasa* as a state of neutral consciousness. It is said to be the natural state of mind from which all the other emotions emerge.
[13] Ammannur Madhava Chakyar, "My Training, My Gurus" in *Sangeet Natak*, (Special issue), no. 111-114, p. 141-146.
[14] Ibid., p. 145-46.
[15] This *Svara-vayu* method in *Kudiyattam* does not have any direct connections to the breathing method I suggest in Chapter 2, the *Siva Svarodaya Shastra*.
[16] T. K. Ramunni Nair, *Natyarcana*, (Calicut: P.K. Brothers, 1955), p. 90-96.
[17] Ammannur Madhava Chakyar, "My Training, My Gurus" in *Sangeet Natak*, (Special issue), no. 111-114, p. 146.
[18] G. Venu, "Swaravayu: A Unique Method of Breath-Control", in *Sruti: Music & Dance Magazine*, issue 125, Feb 1995, p. 45.
[19] Ibid., p. 45.
[20] Yoshi, Oida, *The Invisible Actor*, (London: Methuen, 1997), p. 89-92.
[21] Alison Hodge, *Twentieth Century Actor Training*, (ed.), (London & New York: Routledge, 2000), p. 66.
[22] Ibid., p. 71.
[23] Ibid., p. 22.
[24] Jerzy Grotowski, *Towards a Poor Theatre*, (London: Methuen, 1991), p. 175.
[25] Ibid., p. 176.
[26] Ibid., p. 176
[27] Ibid., p. 117-18.
[28] See Grotowski's comparison, which is elementary and can not expect from a serious researcher. It seems that he is familiar with some breathing exercises in Hatha Yoga but not aware of the deeper understaning and practice of breath in Yoga. See Chapter 2 for more details.
[29] Jacques Lecoq, *The Moving Body: Teaching Creative Theatre*, (London: Methuen, 2000)p. 76.

[30] John Martin, *The Intercultural Performance Handbook,* (London: Routledge, 2004), p. 19-27.
[31] Ibid., p. 34.
[32] I gathered this information in my field research in Kerala from an *Yogi* whom I contacted for *Siddha* Yoga practice. His name is Rajendra *Siddha Yogi* who did not allow me to talk more about him. As he said, Osho also mentioned it in one of his speeches.
[33] Phillip Zarrilli, " On the Edge of A Breath, Looking", in Phillip Zarrilli, (ed.), *Acting (Re)Considered,* (London: Routledge, 1995), p. 180.
[34] Ibid., p. 190.
[35] Ibid., p. 191.
[36] Ibid., p. 191.
[37] Nicolas Núñez, *Anthropocosmic Theatre,*(Amsterdam: Harwood, 1996), p. 131.
[38] Peter Malekin & Ralph Yarrow, *Consciousness, Literature and Theatre: Theory and Beyond,* (London: Macmillan Press, 1997), p. 136.
[39] Ibid., p. 136.
[40] Ibid., p. 136.
[41] Peter Malekin (1999), "Performance and Consciousness as Freedom", in *Performing Arts International,* vol. 1, parts 4, p. 95.
[42] Daniel Meyer-Dinkgräfe, *Consciousness and the Act*, (Frankfurt: Peter Lang, 1996), p. 154.
[43] Cicely Berry, *Voice and the Actor,*(London: Virgin Books, 2000), p. 7
[44] Ibid., p. 18-42.
[45] <http://kh.bu.edu/artwithbraininmind-1/1736.html> (consulted July 12, 2007.
[46] Ibid., p. 76-77.
[47] Daniel Meyer-Dinkgräfe, *Consciousness and the Actor*, (Frankfurt: Peter Lang, 1996). p. 160.
[48] Alison Hodge, *Twentieth Century Actor Training,* (ed.), (London & New York: Routledge, 2000), p. 160.
[49] Ibid., p. 162.

Chapter Four
Breath and Consciousness

Consciousness studies, as an academic discipline, includes a wide range of theoretical investigations across the disciplines of philosophy, neuroscience, cognitive science and psychology, physical and biological sciences and computer science. The word *consciousness* primarily refers to human beings aware of and responsive to their surroundings. Consciousness, in this sense, implies a human being that is conscious of something; the contents of consciousness in turn are based on individual perception and action that come with intuitions and feelings. Consciousness studies, therefore, are engaged in a systematic analysis of essential functions of the mind within the physicality of the body. In theatre, the inner dynamics of production and reception of theatrical meaning and experience are embedded in the mind/body of the actor. That is why consciousness studies is relevant to theatre both in theory and in practice. In recent years, systematic analysis of rituals and non-Western performance forms has benefited from the application of models of consciousness found in the *Advaita Vedanta* philosophy of India. Vedic model of consciousness, proposed by Maharishi Mahesh Yogi, for instance, confirms the existence of higher levels of consciousness beyond the intellect and emotions. He also explained the phenomenon of *pure consciousness*, a concept developed from *Advaita Vedanta* philosophy. The following sections will offer more information about it. The key intention of this chapter is to establish a possible connection between breath, time and consciousness, aiming to argue that the level of consciousness can be altered through systematic application of intentional breathing.

4.1 Consciousness: Early Views

In *The Discovery of the Mind*, German classicist Bruno Snell gives an account of the descriptions of the changes of human personality over the centuries from Homer to Socrates. According to Snell, Homer believed that "the psyche is the force which keeps the human being alive[1] and when the psyche leaves the owner loses consciousness. Homer further believed that consciousness is a force which is separate from the body. Books VI and VII of Plato's *The*

Republic illustrate Platos' contribution to consciousness studies. While discussing the relationship and properties of things, Plato suggests the existence of 'the eye of the mind':

> And do you not know also that although they make use of the visible forms and reason about them, they are thinking not of these, but of the ideals which they resemble; not of the figures which they draw, but of the absolute square and the absolute diameter, and so on—the forms which they draw or make, and which have shadows and reflections in water of their own, are converted by them into images, but they are really seeking to behold the things themselves, which can only be seen with the eye of the mind? (Republic: vi)

Here, Plato establishes the idea of consciousness, metaphorically, through introducing the notion of 'the eye of the mind' which is capable of observing mental content arranged in geometrical forms. He further explains the faculty of understanding "as being intermediate between opinion and reason". Plato, at this stage of his argument, proposes the existence of a state of mind that observes the human cognitive process of logical reasoning and arrives at interpretive opinions, associated with the moments of our understanding of objects and events. This level of mind is beyond reason and opinion, it can also contemplate knowledge.

> I understand you to say that knowledge and being, which the science of dialectic contemplates, are clearer than the notions of the arts, as they are termed, which proceed from hypotheses only: these are also contemplated by the understanding, and not by the senses: yet, because they start from hypotheses and do not ascend to a principle, those who contemplate them appear to you not to exercise the higher reason upon them, although when a first principle is added to them they are cognizable by the higher reason (Republic: vi)

Here, Plato establishes the links between art and consciousness, stating that art is contemplative like knowledge and being when the mimetic element is added onto it. In his analogy of the cave, Plato describes that experiences are copies of real things rather than the things themselves: "…the shadows which he formerly saw are truer than the objects which are now shown to him?"[2] Consciousness, for Plato, is an intermediatory state of mind that operates between reason and opinion and moves naturally beyond rationality of thoughts. As Malekin and Yarrow suggest, "Plato is logically showing the point at which logic collapses."[3] They argue that these traditional models of consciousness, proposed by Homer and Plato, are pre-spatial and pre-temporal and the surface divisions of space-time do not apply to them. Within the Platonic tradition, as they further explain, Plotinus proposed three major modes of consciousness: 1. the everyday waking level which includes "discursive thought and sequential sensory perception". 2. the noetic mode, which is "ontologically prior to differentiated space and time", in which "cognition is a direct uniting with the object, and both subject and object constitute parts that contain the whole" 3. "a merging into timeless infinitude" in which "individual mind, ego, object worlds and subject-object cognition all drop away."[4] Plotinus asserts that the third one is the good one and people should maintain that level of consciousness together with other ordinary states like waking cognition and dreaming experience. Malekin and Yarrow elaborately discuss Plotinus's model of mind in comparison with Indian and oriental models of consciousness, which we will look at in the following section as a recent trend in contemporary consciousness studies.

4.2 Consciousness: Recent Views

Recent explanations of consciousness fall into four broader categories: 1) functionalism 2) dualism 3) eliminativism 4) mysterianism. According to functionalism, the mental states that create consciousness can essentially be defined as complex interactions between different functional processes that are not limited to a particular physical state or physical medium. They can be realized in multiple ways including within non-biological systems like digital computers.[5] Dualist theories of consciousness propose that phenomenal experience occurs in a non-physical place. The 'thinking' (brain) is the non-physical place in Cartesian dualism whereas the phenomenal world is the non-physical place in Reid's natural dualism. Property dualism asserts that mental properties emerge when matter is organized in the appropriate way. Property dualism is a branch of emergent materialism, which is the basis of scientific theories dealing with emergent phenomena.[6] Eliminative materialism is the school of thought that argues for an absolute version of materialism and physicalism with respect to mental entities and mental vocabulary. Eliminative materialists, therefore, believe that consciousness does not exist and what is known as consciousness is the neurophysical functioning of the body. Similarly, they argue that folk psychological concepts such as belief, desire and intention do not have any consistent neurological substrate.[7] The term mysterianism refers to a philosophy that proposes that certain problems like consciousness will never be explained and humans do not have the intellectual ability to understand the problem of consciousness at a scientific level. This position is also known as anti-constructive-naturalism.[8] Panpsychism or panexperientialism is another theoretical model explaining the nature of consciousness. According to this model, consciousness is everywhere, an idea that seems consistent with Eastern metaphysical principles and as a possible solution to an interpretation of quantum physics. Capra, in *The Tao Physics*, observes the parallels between Eastern metaphysics and quantum physics as follows:

> Modern physics… pictures matter not at all as passive and inert, but as being in a continuous dancing and vibrating motion whose rhythmic patterns are determined by the molecular, atomic and nuclear structures. This is also the way in which the Eastern mystics see the material world. They all emphasise that the universe has to be grasped dynamically, as it moves, vibrates and dances; the nature is not in a static, but a dynamic equilibrium. (Capra, 1976, 205)[9]

This view clarifies the kinetic base involved in the existence of nature and the activities of perception and production of meanings, which generate levels of individual consciousness. Capras' view also suggests that consciousness is a process, not a thing. As Jane Roberts observes, consciousness fields produce consciousness particles that in turn become matter and energy. The thought you think and the rock you see, are patterns of consciousness. Consciousness is fundamental pure subjectivity.[10]

One of the recent trends in the studies of consciousness is informed by Sanskrit tradition of India. As Malekin and Yarrow observe, "It is the Vedic tradition of India that has produced the systematic and formulated schematizations of growth in states of consciousness".[11] They discuss a model of consciousness found in the *Mandukya Upanishad* explaining four levels of consciousness: waking, dreaming, sleeping and *Turiya*. "*Turiya* is an underlying unconditioned consciousness which appears limited when reflected through the three contingent states of the individual mind."[12]

Gaudapada and Sankara, the major commentators of *Advaita Vedanta* philosophy of India, consider *Turiya* as the deepest underlying reality of the mind and the "Reality itself."[13] Malekin and Yarrow further explain *Turiya* as an eternal sense of experience:

> *Turiya* is cloaked if the mind is dispersed by attachment to the worlds of objects, but in itself *Turiya* is eternal, so that from the point of view of the relative individual mind *Turiya,* once realised, permeates all the relative states of walking, dreaming and sleeping; in other words, unconditioned awareness accompanies and underlies all walking and dreaming activity and lasts through what would ordinarily be the blackness of deep sleep.[14]

Turiya, the fourth level of consciousness, is understood and explained as a higher level of consciousness alternating 'stillness' with the 'activity' of ordinary levels of consciousness. *Turiya* also suggests a particular level of mind by which the 'stillness' is maintained increasingly during and together with activities; this state of mind is neutral and its experience is highly recommended by various spiritual systems of practice in India as a quality state of individual being because this 'neutral consciousness' will bring some of the crucial strength and qualities which cannot be identified otherwise in an ordinary level of consciousness. Most of India's meditation techniques and related *yogic* practices suggest the ways of achieving this neutral consciousness called *Turiya.* This means that *yogic* practice and meditation techniques are methods to achieve *Turiya* or neutral consciousness through a spatial and temporal shift in the ordinary level of consciousness.

The idea of a spatio-temporal shift in consciousness has succeeded in achieving considerable importance in Malekin and Yarrow's writings. While re-reading Plotinian terms they propose a mode of consciousness which is 'eternal' and also characterised by 'unbounded timelessness'. Malekin conducts a parallel reading between art and spirituality arguing that "[a] trained Indian classical vocalist is a yogi, trained from childhood to produce overtones in the voice conducive to a settling of the mind even during intense enjoyment of the movement of the music."[15] Malekin argues further, in relation to the musician, that "the production of the requisite register can only come from the settled mind of the performer. The settlement is perfect when the outer level of activity flows unimpeded while the inner level of mind remains beyond movement or rest in boundless infinitude."[16] This level of consciousness is beyond subject-object boundaries, which is the union (*Yoga*) of other levels of consciousness. As Malekin suggests, both the artist/performer and the Yogi experience the same level of consciousness that is beyond the time frame set by ordinary activities in the waking and dreaming states. In India, great performers and artist were traditionally regarded as saints. The iconic figure of the dancing Shiva represents two ideas: Shiva the dancer and Shiva the Yogi. In *yogic* terms, Shiva's dancing represents the delight of experiencing, of being within *Turiya,* the consciousness which is timeless or beyond any ordinary sense of time. In the context of theatre, the dancing represents the delight of *rasa*, an experience which is essentially the same as the experience of *Turiya.* In the *Natyasastra,* Bharata introduces a similar concept by saying that the experience of theatre is similar to the experience of *Brahman*, the infinitude in consciousness because the art of theatre has been created by Brahma and Lord Shiva is the first actor.[17] Performance, for Bharata, in this sense, is a means to access the inaccessible, the delight of *rasa*, which is similar to experiencing *Brahman.* This means that performance and meditation are two different psychophysical ways of experiencing the same level of consciousness which exists beyond the spatio-temporal dimensions of the waking and dreaming states of consciousness. Malekin further explains this level of consciousness as the "unbounded silence of infinitude" out of which patterns of sounds and forms emerge in space and time: "form arises in sound and out of this space and time are born."[18] For Malekin, *Turiya* is a state of "unbounded silence of infinitude" and therefore, performance of any kind striving to achieve that level of consciousness is an act of freedom because the actor breaks up subject-object boundaries and the ordinary sense of time-space relations. Waking and dreaming consciousness are bound by the (*karmic*) laws of cause and effect at work in the material world. Finding a place outside of the material world by breaking up the sequence of *karmic* repetition of events and occurrences brings freedom (*mukti*) into individual consciousness. In short, *Turiya* as an altered state of human consciousness, experienced as "unbounded silence of infinitude" that exists beyond the ordinary spatio-temporal relations. Malekin here clearly suggests that a crucial shift is taking place, spatially and temporally, in consciousness when we experience the alteration in consciousness that is *Turiya*. The ordinary individual mode of consciousness, according to Malekin, can be altered through ritual, music and chanting. In other words, rituals, music and chanting can be considered as practical methods through which the individual consciousness can be changed.

Yarrow's concept of 'neutral consciousness' shares Malekin's argument about an alteration of individual consciousness through a shift in spatio-temporality. As he asserts, "consciousness is not a static phenomenon, but a historical process in time."[19] Aesthetic experience is "psychologically and physiologically mediated" and "art is what happens to our bodies and minds—just as "matter" may be explicable in terms of energy transformation also characteristic of consciousness."[20] Yarrow considers consciousness as a psycho-physical quality which functions on various levels in individual cognition. Neutrality becomes a state, distinct from other states of consciousness, "where silence and activity co-exist"; it is the "simplest state of awareness", which "...might be thought of as a psycho-physiological quantum mechanical state of Zero entropy like superconductivity."[21] Yarrow argues that this is not an abstract state but "a fulcrum condition central to symbolic utterances of all kinds"; the application of mask and movement in training explains the physical condition of this level of consciousness in theatrical terms. As he explains, the mask creates a 'self' and a 'mirror self' in the actor and the actor perceives the 'real-self' and the 'mirror-self' as separate, but connected. Seeing through a mask, in this sense, gives the actor the possibility to achieve a witnessing quality of consciousness by staying in the space between herself and her projected masked self. As Yarrow puts it:

> Understanding it in physical terms helps to clarify that we are not talking about an abstract idea but a phenomenon which, because it is the minimal point of activity, is accessible via any efficient means of moving from states of mind and body where there is a more diverse "scatter" of energy to those where it is more subtly compacted.[22]

Two major assumptions can be derived here from in Yarrows' investigations of consciousness: 1. Neutral consciousness is the place where silence and activity co-exist 2. Neutral consciousness is an altered state of consciousness, which is a psycho-physical condition of the mind and the body. In addition to this, Yarrow further establishes the links between quantum physics and consciousness, arguing that *altered consciousness* suggests "a merging of one state …into a more expanded version."[23] Quantum theory recognizes that particles manifest themselves as distinct quanta of energy at different frequencies and there are non-localized waves, which themselves can be derived from the "plenum" or vacuum state, which contains potential energy. According to Yarrow, to apply this to consciousness clearly suggests that a neutral or potential state of consciousness is categorically parallel to non-localized waves emerging from the vacuum, which is characteristically distinct from the already known modes of consciousness modes like waking and dreaming.[24]

Yarrow emphasizes a transcendent quality "reflecting in the operation of consciousness which embraces and organizes all the diverse parts or perspectives."[25] He explains the links between consciousness and space-time by looking at the process of reading: as in the quantum view of physical reality, "characters and events can be seen as processes in space-time rather than isolated phenomena…and [It is possible to] view the text as a generative set of relations rather than a closed phenomenon."[26] Thus, consciousness is transformational energy" operating within the basis of mind-body by using space-time as transformational tools. This means that any change taking place on the level of consciousness includes a significant shift in the relations of space-time. Waking and dreaming, in this sense, will have distinct space-time associations in our experience and *Turiya* or neutral consciousness go beyond the level of ordinary understanding of time. Malekin's 'timeless infinitude' and Yarrow's 'silence co-existing with activity' suggest the implications of the transformational characteristics of consciousness, which are understood as "awareness of its own nature as potential", a form of energy united with matter as "energy-filled void."[27] This is known as unity consciousness in the *Vedanta* model of mind proposed in terms of Vedic Science and Vedic Psychology by Maharishi Mahesh Yogi; a comprehensive description of this model is available in Meyer-Dinkgräfe (2005).

According to Meyer-Dinkgräfe, Vedic Psychology describes four higher levels of human consciousness in addition to waking, dreaming and sleeping. What Malekin and Yarrow describe in terms of *Turiya* is thus further differentiated, as follows:[28]

Pure Consciousness: It is the fourth state of human development besides waking, dreaming and sleeping. As such it is the basis of more expressed level of awareness defined as the "over all multilevel functioning of consciousness."[29] This is the level of "timeless infinitude" (Malekin). *Cosmic consciousness*, a fifth state, in which pure consciousness is experienced as co-existing with waking, dreaming and sleeping. In this state of consciousness, pure consciousness or the Self witnesses the activities of waking, dreaming and sleeping. Meyer-Dinkgräfe offers a description of how this state manifests in individual experience by quoting David W. Orme-Johnson from the collected scientific research papers on the Transcendental Meditation Programme:

> Often during dreaming I am awake inside, in a very peaceful, blissful state. Dreams come and go, thoughts about the dreams come and go, but I remain in a deeply peaceful state, completely separate from the dreams and the thoughts. My body is asleep and inert, breathing goes on regularly and mechanically, and inside I am just aware that I am.[30]

The next stage of development, according to Vedic Psychology is *refined cosmic consciousnesses*. In cosmic consciousness, pure consciousness is permanently experienced together with waking, dreaming and sleeping. In refined cosmic consciousness, this level is maintained along with "the maximum value of perception of the environment... [and] perception and feeling reach their most sublime level."[31] The philosopher Fichte describes the experience of this level of consciousness as follows:

> ...and the universe appears before my eyes clothed in a more glorious form. The dead inert mass which only filled up space, has vanished: and in its place there flows onward, with the rushing music of mighty waves, an endless stream of life and power and action, which issues from the original source of all life.[32]

Unity consciousness is the ultimate level of human development according to Vedic Psychology and in this state of consciousness "the field of pure consciousness is directly perceived as located at every point in creation" and therefore, every point in creation is raised to the

...status of pure consciousness.[33] The duality between 'relative' and the 'absolute' in the perception of things in life does no longer exist in this state of consciousness. The distinctions between knowledge, knower and knowing will be united into an absolute sense of awareness. As the *Bhagadvad Gita* describes unity consciousness: "The Yogi who is united in identity with the all-pervading, infinite consciousness, and see unity everywhere, beholds the Self present in all beings, and all beings as assumed in the Self."[34] Unity consciousness, as the highest level of human consciousness, is described in various *Upanishads,* the *Bhagavad Gita* and classical Indian texts of *Yoga* including *Yoga-Vasishta.* Patanjali's term *samadhi* and *Advaita Vedanta's* term *Turiya* refer to a state of individual consciousness explained in unity consciousness.

Pure consciousness is the result of a distinct perception of space and time. When the ordinary perception of time and space are modified, what exists in the experience of an individual is the "timeless" and "spaceless."[35] Malekin and Yarrow share the idea of going beyond ordinary space-time parameters in the experience of individual consciousness by presenting concepts like "silence co-exists with activity" and "timeless infinitude". I can summarise, from the writings of Malekin, Yarrow and Meyer-Dinkgräfe, as follows:

1. Altered states of consciousness exist in individual experience, which are named and described differently under different systems of thought. Hence, terms such as *Samadhi* and *pure consciousness* refer to the same experience of consciousness. The concept of *Turiya* also includes the concept of pure consciousness, although not on its own, but in relation to, and experienced together with, waking, dreaming and sleeping (see 5 below).

2. This field of pure consciousness exists beyond the ordinary perception of day-to-day time-space parameters.

3. Modification of space-time parameters can result in the experience of "timeless infinitude".

4. Pure consciousness is an undivided form of awareness in which all forms of duality between subject and object, and meaning and cognition submerge into a unity of self awareness: nothing exists here except the existence of Self at end.

5. Just as pure consciousness on its own is characterised by a space-time configuration that is different from the space-time configuration in waking, or dreaming or sleeping on their own, the coexistence, in terms of Vedic Psychology, of waking, dreaming and sleeping with pure consciousness in cosmic, refined cosmic and unity consciousness, equally represents different space-time configurations. Changes of space-time configurations may serve to bring about the experience of any of these higher states of consciousness.

In short, consciousness generally emerges in a phenomenological relationship with different modalities and qualities of perception. There is also a kind of consciousness which seems to operate 'outside' of this perceptual modalities as 'witness' to any phinomenological situation. This level is nornally understood as extended or altered level of consciousness. How far this extension of consciousness is associated with a cessation of breath is the question that I am going to address in the following sections. Cessation of breath always underpinnes and conditions a retention or suspension of psychophysiological activities. It is clear in the descriptions of the above writers that individual consciousness can be modified by modifying time space parameters. In the following sections I will look at the scope and potential of human breathing investigationg how changes in the modalities of breathing change the level of consciousness. I will also suggest that breath is an effective tool to modify individual perception of time-space in experiencing the extended 'witnessing' level of consciousness. I will also look at *santarasa* as an example of the implication of breath and consciousness in performance.

4.3 Time and Consciousness

Consciousness can be understood as patterns of spatio-temporal relations. Being conscious, in this sense, means that being consciousness of something that exists in space and time. Cognition, therefore, is a spatio-temporal activity extended to the present infinite. Consciousness is thus a kinetic experience, and kinetic consciousness, fundamentally, is a "stream of present" as Husserl would describe it. The link between modalities of time, space and consciousness in relation to cognition is the fundamental theme running across several strands in contemporary philosophical thinking like phenomenology, hermeneutics and deconstruction. What is fundamental to the process of human cognition is the act of restoring of a 'past' time into a 'present' by using 'memory' as a tool. The moment which is *past* can be *memorised* in order to cognate. Memory as an act of meaning operates in the field of a subjective movement that goes back to the recorded impressions of past events and comes forward to a present in which what is carried forward is re-cognised. This essential nature of the dynamics of human cognition operates in time, in the kinetic modalities of time. Repetition, as a philosophical concept explains this fundamental aspect of human consciousness. I will briefly explain the concept here to establish links between time and consciousness, which will also set the background of the discussion of breath in the following sections.

4.3.1 Repetition and Consciousness

Repetition, as a movement-related philosophical view, is crucial to literary and philosophical enquiries because the term explains the nature of meaning and consciousness in terms of human cognitive processes. Kierkegaard established the term *repetition* in 1843 in his work *Repetition: An Essay in Experimental Psychology* as an important philosophical category. *Repetition* and *recollection* are the same movement but in opposite directions: what has been recollected is repeated backwards, whereas the 'real' repetition is recollected forwards. *Repetition* as a philosophical term influenced later developments of the theories of meaning in Western philosophical traditions, especially in the post-phenomenological strands including hermeneutics and deconstruction. As Melberg explains, "the temporal device of *repetition* is a paradoxical movement between past and present…and time as a process of past into present."[36] Repetition as a textual device of reading refers to a kind of movement back and forth that goes on between different parts of the text, between its irony and its pathos, between two characters of the narration, between the narrator and his/her object and between the text and its reader. Melberg, in his attempt to examine the implications of *repetition* in theories of representation extensively analysed the concept of *mimesis*, discussed by Plato and Aristotle. Melberg argues that Plato uses the word *mimesis* in a primarily visual context, as a visual image related to imitation.

In the dialogue on creation, *Timaeus*, Plato has the title character discuss the mimetic relation between image, imitation and time. Timaeus states that the world we live in has been created in the greatest similarities to the creator himself (29 E-30D). The metaphors used in this philosophical debate on creation are particularly visual and give the impression of the first creator as a kind of pictorial artist. The analogy of the cave in the seventh book of the Republic is another example that Plato's philosophy is based on sight or has a visual orientation. Melberg's analysis of Platonic *mimesis* culminates with the logical problems of time described by Timaeus when he says that creation was made in relation to the principle of similarity. It was not possible, says Timaeus, for the creator to make the image that is our world eternal and constant; he adds that the world carries traces of its constant origin as a "moving image of eternity" (37D) and what we call time is nothing but an image *(eikona)* of eternity (37D). As a visual proof, Timaeus gives the example of stars as the eternal repetition of the same circuit: "this very world must be as similar as possible to the absolute being that can be grasped by the mind and imitating its eternal nature" (39 DE). Melberg considers these lines remarkable because they are the only ones where Plato discusses time-change-movement in terms of *mimesis* as he argues "*mimesis* here becomes repetition."[37]

Mimesis is an equally important concept for Aristotle in his *Poetics*. According to Gerald F. Else, Aristotle not only changes the Platonic evolution of *mimesis*, but also changes the meaning of the concept, when he says: "[it] ends up meaning almost the exact opposite of what Plato had meant by it."[38] Aristotle defines the new function of *mimesis* with the concepts of *mythos* and *praxis* in the sixth chapter of the *Poetics* as "an imitation of an action". It is primarily the *mythos*, the plot, which is the imitation of the action. *Mythos* is the "structure of events" that Aristotle calls "the soul of the tragic art" (50 a 38/39). *Praxis* is rather one event that is "serious, complete and has bulk" (47b 25). In addition, in the seventh chapter we get the famous definition of *praxis* as an action "which is complete and a whole and has a certain magnitude". It is an action, furthermore, with "beginning, middle and end" (50b 24-27). Melberg provides a concise summary of this argument as follows:[39]

1. Aristotle's *mimesis* is defined by *mythos* and *praxis*, which bring the concept close to areas of time and action – in contrast to Platonic *mimesis* which is closer to image, imagination and imitation.

2. *Mythos* is a concept of order, which makes it possible to view literary works as structured wholes.

3. *Praxis* refers to already structured events or chains of events, which can be perceived as meaningful and answering a purpose.

As Paul Ricoeur observes, *mimesis* appears to be a temporal concept in Aristotle as the "lived temporal experience."[40] In fact, Ricoeur's analysis of *mimesis* was a reply against its own illusionism as well as against deconstructive criticism of the "closure of representation". Ricoeur intended to treat *mimesis* as a process, which he calls *mimesis 1, mimesis 2 and mimesis 3. Mimesis* needs something to imitate and here Ricoeur refers to Aristotle's key expression that the poem is the imitation of an action. *Mimesis*, therefore, pre-supposes a generally accepted pre-conception of what an action is; this action is then transplanted into a text and finally realised by the reader. Here Ricoeur has given greater emphasis on the act of reading as a process or a movement from 'prefigured' world to 'transfigured' world through 'configured' textual world. Unlike many phenomenologists who relate *mimesis* to the visible world, Ricoeur relates it to action and says that the phenomenal world is the world of movement, time and change; imaginary mimetic activity is essentially connected with repetition and therefore, time. Again in the words of Ricoeur, "time becomes human time to the extent that it is organised after the manner of a narrative: narrative, in turn, is meaningful to the extent that it portrays the features of temporal experience."[41] Hence, repetition is an action, which gives certain consciousness, knowledge and experience mediated by memory. Kierkegaard, the philosopher of repetition says since we can not recover our lost beginning and cannot survive beyond our inevitable end, the reenactment of life in literature entails genuine repetition – a "repetition properly so called is recollected forward."[42] Every re-enactment, whether in literature or performance is a repetition in order to make the inaccessible appear through a multiple and complex operation of time, action and memory. Both reading and performance are re-enactments of situations in 'real' life, and *repetition*, as a critical term explains this process of the nature of the production of meaning. Memory works as a key tool in this process of repetition or re-enactment bringing time and action together. Recollection, in this sense, is a temporal act which brings actions, reactions and emotions into play. Repetition, in this manner, establishes the links between time and consciousness; consciousness is a temporal experience operating on the basis of a subjective movement, which is going back to memory and forth to re-cognition.

In both the writings of Derrida and Deleuze we see repetition as an underpinning concept reinforcing a radical philosophical thinking based on the temporal dialectics of presence and meaning that deconstructed the 'stigma of Western thinking' since Plato. Derrida describes the nature and function of meaning in terms of *presence* as the structure of repetition. As he explains, the sign in general has its own origin in repetition, in a "primordial structure of repetition". 'Presence' derives from the constant perceptual re-occurrence of signs and therefore, presence must be derived from repetition. Derrida emphasises that the identification or the meaning of a particular sign is derived from its re-appearance and therefore, mediated by and through memory.

It is highly useful at this stage to look at Foucault's observations on repetition to understand the psycho-physical implications of the term. While commenting on Deleuze's intellectual contribution to the history of Western thought, Foucault examines two aspects of the nature of cognition:[43]

1) the methodologies of the recent past that attempt to conceptualise the nature of being
2) the nature of an event.

Foucault examines the nature of event and says that "event is not a concept" but strictly a "temporal force" which only exists in the present time. The occurrence of an event cannot be controlled or defined by any methodological programmes. An event might occur without our being able to define the nature or consequences of what is taking place. An event can be narrated only after its occurrence. An event therefore, is an active process that takes place in the structural dimensions of space and temporality. In his reassessment of the philosophical methodologies of the recent past, Foucault argues that neither neo-positivism nor classical phenomenology can explain this dynamics of temporalization involved in an event. According to Foucault, Deleuze's contribution to contemporary philosophy is a methodology, a methodology which helps to understand the nature of temporality involved in our understandings of meaning and consciousness. This methodology is called repetition; it is a state of always being in the "present infinitive". So, each moment of *being* is the being continuously in the present time.

An event is the smallest unit of time that is taking place in time. It is also the smallest unit of knowledge or sense of being. In other words, cognition or the sense of being is the result of the process of a series of occurrences of body, language and thoughts in the present time. Deleuze further argues that unlike representation, which is conceptual, *repetition* is a psycho-physical phenomenon, embedded in moments in the present time and space. Deleuze explained repetition by identifying two recurring infinite elements that operate in the process of making sense of the world:

1) Remembering and recognition
2) Memory and self-consciousness

Each moment of recognition is the movement of repetition of *physis* and *psyche*, the pure force of the psycho-physical movement in time and space.

Deleuze's repetition however, represents a particular tradition of philosophy and the continuation of the idea of the temporal notion of philosophical thinking in the West presented by a group of philosophers like Kierkegaard, Nietzsche, Heidegger, Freud, Marx and Derrida. The temporal dimension of human existence is the most fascinating perspective "chosen for the interpretation of being" (Heidegger 1999, 206) by these philosophers. As Heidegger elucidates, *time* as a basic concept and an essential 'perspective governing' the conditions of being has "remained essentially undeveloped" from the beginnings of Western philosophy until Aristotle. Heidegger further explains *time* as "the actual moment" of *now*: "past is the *no-longer-now* [and] future is the *not-yet-now* [and therefore] being in the sense of already-thereness (presence) became the perspective for the determination of time" (Heidegger 1999, 206). Derrida admits the fact that the concepts of 'temporalization' and 'displacement' are already explained by Nietzsche and Freud as "active" moments in metaphysics as well as in psychoanalysis as the function of thought and unconscious.[44] According to Deleuze, the turning point in Freud was a decisive moment in which he incorporated *time* in his *Beyond the Pleasure Principles* as phenomenon of repetition.[45] Time is everywhere: in language, in reading and in all doing. Time is in consciousness and in our knowledge of the world. The whole question of *being* and the entire material existence of the world are clearly marked in this passage of *time*. No time is no meaning and no being. The development of critical theories in recent years, particularly the terms *difference*, *theatricality* and *performativity*, is informed by this psycho-physical movement in philosophical thinking known as repetition.

4.4 Breath and Consciousness

The previous section has demonstrated how time and consciousness are interconnected and how the temporal stream of consciousness reflects on cognitive processes in various forms of representation including theatre practice. Breath flows parallel to the temporal stream of consciousness, and breath, therefore, is the physical counterpart of time realised in the human organism. No breathing means no time and therefore, no being. As Irigaray asserts, "To live-to breathe: to become-to change/alter"[46] and therefore, breath, being the basis of human activity, is fundamental to human cognition.

4.4.1 Breathing and Being: A New Philosophy

If the psychic impulses (memory and re-cognition) and their physical motivations are considered as the repetitive nature of human existence, is there anything in the psycho-physicality of the human organism, which activates and reinforces the process of repetition? Heidegger asks the same question in his *Introduction to Metaphysics* as "what is the temporal extension of human life…"[47] and he makes a crucial point in this context stating that breath, as a movement, is the temporal extension of human life, which activates and reinforces the psychic impulses of memory and re-cognition and its physical motivations, in order to manifest our sense of Being in time. Breath is time in this sense, and no presence and its re-cognition are possible without the constant bi-polar movement of breathing. Breath is present time and also the presence of time. What is being grasped in the present time as presence is mediated by a definite mode of time through nostril operations. This perpetual movement of respiration, as the definite mode of present time, is the basis of the *play* of presence and absence, meaning and void and memory and forgetfulness.

Irigaray goes further saying that if breath is considered as the temporal extension of Being, there is no Being without breathing. Air is always there, although we tend to forget it. It is an unrecognised "place of all presence and absence" and "no presence is possible without air."[48] The place of no breath is the place of disappearance. Air plays between presence and absence, between life and death, between significations and their perception; and between representation and its cognition. This imperceptible materiality of air is the "forgotten *material mediation* of the *logos*."[49] Irigaray suggests that the air element is the mediation of all reflections including perception, language, thoughts, imagination and the faculty of action. In the particular context of signification and meaning, Irigaray asserts that air is the invisible *other*, which is irreducible and without which there is no movement between perception and cognition. The flow of air is the passage of time, and therefore, the producer of consciousness. The flow of air is the flow of the language, and therefore, the producer of meaning.

Derrida, in *Dissemination*, goes beyond the perpetual repetition of textual significations arguing that 'air' is the source of all appearance and that it hovers *between* desire and fulfilment, perpetration and remembrance. Air acts *between* fire and flames, and inside and outside. No air is disappearance. Thus, "[a]ir means, this *is-trying-to-say* that," which means that being is always in the "present infinitive", and this obviously includes "the temporal extension of Being" and the "temporality of consciousness". Derrida extends this understanding of the role of breath in Being by saying that "what is called 'present' is described as represented....but [this representation] is filled with Air." What we see in both Derrida and Irigaray is the act of thinking, of meaning, representation and consciousness, in terms of breathing. Repetition is explained by Deleuze as a psycho-physical movement: the psychic movement of recollection and re-cognition; and the physical movement of fulfilment of desire. Both these movements are based on the invisible existence and the dynamics of breath. Hence, the constant repetition of the presence and our simultaneous reflections on it as "Being" are manifested through the repetition of breath. Here, I can see the emergence of a new philosophical thinking in Derrida and Irigaray: the philosophy of breathing.

4.4.2 Breath and Representation: Artaud's Divine Theatre

Artaud has discussed the role of breath in theatrical representation linking breath into theatrical meaning and experience. Artaud's concept of cruelty emphasises the idea of a *desire*, the desire for always being-in-present. This *desire* is the psycho-physical urge to be in the present, to be in consciousness: the underlying energy to all the emotional and cognitive processes. The failure of theatre, according to Artaud, is forgetting this *desire*, this temporal dimension that creates movement, gestures, sounds and other physical appearances relating to the body. Therefore, theatre is a continuous process and a vibrant movement in space and time that can not be preserved or regained.

Artaud called it the *magical act*. It is *magical* because it is movement which cannot be captured in frozen time: the present transforms into another present, not into future. Artaud's theatre in this sense, "…is a passionate overflowing, a frightful transfer of forces from body to body"[50] and breath was a new means for Artaud's theatre of exploring the "overflowing" of the "frightful transfer of forces" from body to body and from body to its unknown fields of consciousness. However, Artaud left no clear proof of any system of practice though he asserts that "every mental movement, every feeling, every leap in human affectivity has an appropriate breath."[51] However, breathing and consciousness were the major issues that Artaud was trying to articulate by saying that "breathing accompanies feeling and the actor can penetrate this feeling."[52] The key issue here is, knowing the mechanisms of which breathing accompanies which feeling and Artaud, therefore, provides a list of six main breathing combinations between *neuter, feminine* and *masculine*, stating that emotions have a strong base in various patterns of breathing.[53] Below are the six combinations Artaud proposes:

Neuter – Masculine – Feminine
Neuter – Feminine – Masculine
Masculine – Neuter – Feminine
Feminine – Neuter – Masculine
Masculine – Feminine – Neuter
Feminine – Masculine – Neuter

What Artaud was trying to explain was what *Yoga* identifies as the three pathways of human respiration, left, middle and right. These three nostril modes are further categorised according to the qualities that Artaud identifies as well: left – feminine, middle – neuter and right – masculine.[54] Artaud proposes the existence of a seventh state of breath, which is higher than the remaining six modes of breathing. That seventh state unites "the revealed and the unrevealed through the portals of a higher *guna*, the state of *sattva*."[55] *Guna* means the quality and *Sattva* suggests an extended level of experience, which is beyond our daily senses of the world. Meyer-Dinkgräfe offers a clear demonstration of these two terms from the perspective of Vedic psychology:

> The entire creation consists of the interplay of the three gunas (...) born of prakriti or nature. The process of evolution is carried on by these three gunas. Evolution means creation and its progressive development, and at its basis lies activity. Activity needs rajo-guna to create a spur, and it needs sato-guna and tamo-guna to uphold the direction of the movement....For any process to continue, there have to be steps in that process, and each stage, however small in time and space, needs a force to maintain it and another force to develop it into a new shape.[56]

Tamo-guna leads to stagnation and sufferings and *sattva-guna* refers to *sat*, the 'eternal quality' attached to pure consciousness. According to Artaud breath acts as a point of transformation between daily and extra-daily consciousness, between *tamo-guna* and *sattva-guna.* As Artaud suggests, divine theatre can be discovered by "using breathing's hieroglyphics..."[57] Artaud's concept of divine theatre suggests that in theatrical communication the actors engage in systematic breathing exercises to achieve a higher state of consciousness—Artaud uses the term *sattva* in this context. Although Artaud does not seem to have further developed his ideas in practice, I can see close links between these ideas and *Siddha Yoga*. In both the idea of the existence of extended levels of consciousness is conceptualised as the result of a particular way or mode of breathing that goes beyond the ordinary levels of nostril breathing. It is internalised breathing, which is known as *Gati* in *Siddha Yoga* and I will explain this in the following section under *Restoration of Breath.*

Similar to Stanislavski's *rays of energy*[58] Artaud's *Divine Theatre* suggests strong indications of the integration of breath in acting, with the aim of pushing the actor beyond the conventional psychological framework of acting. Stanislavski and Artaud hold similar views on breath:

1) Breath is the vital source of non-verbal physical communication

2) Breath is the key dynamic element working between daily and extra-daily consciousness by uniting the *revealed* and the *unrevealed* into an extended level of consciousness.

3) Breath, through a systematic practice, helps integrate actor's body and mind in such a way that they can communicate through *rays of energy* in the form of psychic radio waves.

According to Stanislavski's concept of the 'rays of energy' breathing is the most effective tool in working with the consciousness of the actor. Stanislavski's and Artaud's attempts of considering breath as a powerful tool and bringing it into their theory and theatre practice seem to be highly relevant to the current discussions of theatre because they introduce consciousness-related training and theory into theatre practice in the West. Stanislavski introduced breath into a consciousness-related actor training by introducing 'rays of energy' and Artaud further expanded the idea theoretically in order to create a philosophical ground appropriate for the kind of theatre practice he wished to introduce.

In the previous section, Irigaray, in a philosophical context, says that the flow of air is the passage of time, and therefore, the producer of consciousness; and the flow of air is the flow of language and therefore, the producer of meaning. By asserting this Irigaray introduces air as an epistemological category by which the production of meaning and consciousness in language can be explained. In a theatrical performance situation, Stanislavski and Artaud consider breath as a potential source of non-verbal physical communication. Unlike through language, for Stanislavski and Artaud, meaning and consciousness in a performance situation is produced through non-verbal psychophysical animations which is supported and reinforced by the inner dynamics of actor's breathing. Beckett's *Acts Without Words*, rasa acting and other physical mimetic movements found in *Kudiyattam* and *Kathakali* can be analysed in this context. In a following section, I will look at the implications of breath in *santarasa*, analysing how breath works psychophysically in the process of creating non-verbal theatrical meaning. However, breath is conceived in both philosophy and theatre as the basis of all meaning and consciousness experienced through language, visibility, appearance, human actions and voice. In both philosophy and theatre, breath is understood as the movement of temporality. It functions as the basis of all the psycho-physical actions in the body that form the basis of the fundamental phenomenon of being, which includes the act of representation and all other discursive means of human communication. In this section we have been looking at and establishing possible links between time and consciousness, and breath and consciousness presented both in philosophy and performance. In the following section, we will look at the philosophical and spiritual dimensions of breathing, presented in Indian systems of thought and practice, linking breath into consciousness and beyond.

4.4.3 *Kāla*: Time and Beyond through Breath

Indian thought has presented a wide range of concepts related to time, movement and consciousness. The term *Kala* refers to time and the non-dualistic school of Kashmir Saivism with its various designations and sub-schools has placed special emphasis on the links between breath and time. The *Svacchanda Tantra* defines time as two-fold: solar and spiritual.[59] Time based on the movement of the astral bodies is gross external time (*Sthula)*, which is solar, and spiritual time is subtle (*suksma*) and related to the movement of the vital air in the body (*prāna*). Abhinavagupta, the 9th century commentator and exponent of Kashmir Saivism says in his *Tantraloka:*

> The whole experience of time (*Kala*) is established in the vital energy of breath (*prana*). The vital energy depends on vibration (*spanda*), vibration rests in the void, and the void in consciousness (*cit*). Therefore, the whole universe is based on consciousness.[60]

Abhinavagupta established the link between breath and consciousness directly and profoundly as the fundamental concept of Kashmir Saivism. Here consciousness means the absolute and timeless consciousness, which evolves in the void. A subtle vibration evolves from the void, which is the source of movement. Time is well connected with movement here and the source of movement is found in the rousing of consciousness as vibrative energy. Abhinavagupta defines vibration (*spandana*) as the fundamental quality of the emergence of the universe from which air and consciousness evolve. Vibration is the subtle movement that causes all the physical manifestations of motion or animation. *Spanda* is the subtle rise of energy which then manifests as the vital air (*prana*). According to Abhinavagupta, consciousness first evolves into vital energy or breath: *prāksamvit prane parinatā*.[61] This movement of the vital air is the source of the expansion of time, according to Kashmir Saivism and time is thus understood as the vibration of consciousness manifest in breath. This understanding of breath is also applicable to microcosmic manifestation, to the creation, maintenance and dissolution of the universe:

> Thus the creation and dissolution of the world are dependent on the vital energy, which in its turn depends on consciousness, and pure consciousness without an object is the...Supreme.[62]

While investigating the relativity of time by describing the experience of time in dream and in sleep, Abhinavagupta asserts that in *Samadhi* there is correspondence between cosmic and microcosmic time, between inbreath and outbreath, between sun and moon and between creation and dissolution. Abhinavagupta devotes the sixth chapter of his *Tantraloka* to the spiritual process called "the way of Time", *kālādhvan*, which incorporates the processes of breath with units and divisions of time. The concept of 'way' (*adhvan*) refers to a process in time as well as a practice on breath. At various points, in the *Tantraloka*, Abhinavagupta alludes to the existence of a breath-related practice in Kashmir Saivism by referring to 'inbreath' and 'outbreath', and 'sun' and 'moon'. Bettina Bäumer further demonstrates that in Abhinavagupta's views on breath, time and consciousness, time and breath are correlatives both in manifestation and withdrawal. The process of "swallowing time" is a process of controlling, observing and sublimating breath. The differentiation between subject and object ceases only when time is thus "swallowed" through breath. "The aim consists therefore, in perceiving the entire temporal way (*adhvan*) in the appearance of one breath..."[63] Abhinavagupta suggests that "the Yogi whose awareness is sharpened by the practice of concentration is able to divide his out-breath and in-breath (*aran* and *apana)*, significantly called sun and moon, into minute units, which are equated with periods of cosmic time."[64] Abhinavagupta suggests that the Yogi can combine his outbreath and inbreath in one moment in his mouth. This act of the integration of breath causes the disappearance of the outer flow of the air through the nostrils. This is the act of internalising breathing and the secret of the limiting and dispersing factor of breath is interconnected in conjunction with the sense of time. The disappearance of breath through internalisation is the disappearance of time. The internalisation operates through a 'gap' located in between outbreath and inbreath. In these 'gaps' time as movement ceases to function. The gap between breaths is thus the gateway to experiencing infinity. Abhinavagupta considered breath as an effective tool to achieve this state beyond time because the individual sense of ordinary time can be altered through altering one's own breathing.

In the *Tantraloka*, Abhinavagupta describes the *Kaladhvan* or "way of Time" thus:

> The Yogi who practices this (voluntary) movement of breath devours it. The gradual withdrawal of breath is the state of the absorption of Time (*kālasamkarsana*) and when this happens, the one pure consciousness shines in its fullness, due to the elimination of the differentiation of knowledge. Thus, since no new movement of breath arises, the differentiation of knowledge does not occur, which is generated by the differentiation of time. Knowledge, in fact, is not fragmented due to the differentiation of the knowable (objects), just like one who is on top of a mountain (and who sees all things at one glance), but rather due to the differentiation of time. In its subtle form this is called the moment. The limit of its subtlety is knowledge, which is precisely the moment (*ksana*).[65]

When this movement of breath stands still, in this way, Time itself ceases and at that moment pure consciousness shines forth without duality in consciousness. We see similar descriptions of this specific breath-related practice in various *Upanishads* described in Chapter two. Abhinavagupta uses the *yogic* metaphors of sun and moon for right and left nostril modes as well as for inbreath and outbreath. There is no evidence of any practice of this kind to be found in other spiritual traditions in India except *Restoration of Breath*, a meditation technique proposed by the *Siddha Yoga* tradition of South India.

4.5 Restoration of Breath

In this chapter, I have so far introduced, in the areas of contemporary critical and philosophical thinking in the West, the links between time and consciousness and their further interconnections with breath. Considering breath as a category of meaning and consciousness is an emerging area of interest and enquiry in the Western philosophical thinking aiming to identify 'Air' as the place of the birth of the phenomenon of *Being* experienced through language, visibility, appearance, human actions and voice. Aristotle dedicated a volume to breath exploring and enquiring into its presocratic roots. For Heidegger, breath is "the temporal extension" of *Being*. Artaud's theatricality is non-representational, and is firmly rooted in the actor's breathing. Following these views and assumptions about breath, leading figures in contemporary Western philosophical thinking, like Jacques Derrida and Luce Irigaray investigate the phenomenon of breath in order to explain the nature of human consciousness. Derrida's 'Air' is the source of the linguistic temporality of ever present textual meanings, but Irigaray goes beyond this linguistic split onto the level of "the origin of the autonomous existence". By considering breath as a new category of philosophical thinking, both Derrida and Irigaray represent a crucial epistemological shift in the West. However, what is missing in this fascinating philosophical thinking is a system that explains the ways in which breath functions in the psycho-physicality of human embodiment in order to understand, consider and establish nostril operations as a category of human cognition. The question I would like to ask here is this: are there any systems of knowledge which offer substantial understanding of the role of breath in the development of individual consciousness.

While there are numerous practises of meditation and *Yoga* that have their origins in India, those relating specifically to using breath as a tool for developing altered states of consciousness are rare. They are kept hidden from the general public for ethical reasons: these techniques are very powerful, with an immediate impact on the body of anyone who practises them. The *Siddha Yoga* tradition is an unusual combination of Saivite spirituality and the practical knowledge of *yogic* breathing techniques of ancient India passed down through a lineage of *Siddhas*. *Siddha Yoga* cannot be reduced to a canon of textual or oral resources, or a fixed set of teachings, though it certainly makes use of texts and teachings. It is purely a practice-based approach, the practice based on breath. The word *Siddha* means the one who attained *siddhi*, or extraordinary powers. Thus the word *Siddha* means the person who has attained or accomplished these powers. *Siddha Yoga* of South India offers a clear system through which we can understand the dynamics of breath in the development of altered states of consciousness. The method in question is called *Restoration of Breath.*

The restoration of breath is a practice-related term. On one level, it explains the ways in which certain performative qualities like psycho-physical energy level, concentration, balance, neutrality and focus could be achieved in the body through training. On another level, it clarifies the existence of the higher states of human consciousness experienced within the body. Both of these can be explored through some specific modes of nostril operations and through the internalisation of breathing. The restoration of breath is a technique and a breath-related practice through which one can totally internalize the respiratory function in order to explore physical and mental presence in training and performance.

According to *Siddha Yoga*, the human respiratory system operates through three paths: left, right and middle. The operating nostril changes intermittently from left to right and right to left during any period of twenty-four hours and in each persistent changeover breath stays in the middle path. The interplay between these three paths of breathing maintains the entire psycho-physical balance of the human organism and therefore, understanding the ways in which breath is controlled and manipulated within the system will offer a perfect control over the whole psycho-physical system. Many of the crucial physiological and psychological experiences of the body from sexual orgasm to birth and death are profoundly interconnected with the dynamics of breath.

The right nostril, being solar or heating in character increases acidic secretions, whereas the left nostril, being lunar or cooling increases alkaline secretions. Therefore, the nostril operations automatically change according to the chemical level of the body in order to maintain the psycho-physical balance. The nostrils influence the body chemistry in different ways. Both the right and the left nostrils are connected with the opposite sides of the cerebral hemispheres and the olfactory lobe. Moreover, the nose is in direct contact with the hypothalamus by its link with the olfactory lobe of the brain. The hypothalamus regulates body temperature, which influences the mental processes and emotional states. The hypothalamus is a part of the limbic system and that part of the brain associated with emotions and motivations. Nostrils, by means of the process of respiration, are connected with neuromotor responses and therefore, with the autonomic nervous system. These neuromotor responses influence the hemispheres of the brain and activate their chemical functions. Neurotransmitters are the brain's chemical messengers and they influence all body functions, including temperature, blood pressure, hormone levels and regular circadian rhythms. It is clear from this medical explanation that human breathing is related to the entirety of psycho-physical being. *Siddha Yoga* offers some specific techniques by which you can change the nostril operations at any moment of time to maintain the energy level of the day. One example of this follows: Sit in a comfortable position, cross-legged and then hold your both toes in a specific sitting position and pull your toes in both sides. You can open your both nostrils by this technique. This nostril mode is called middle path. There is a large hidden territory of knowledge and practice based on these nostril operations.[66]

This middle path is normally understood as the source of vital energy and sometimes more than that. Middle path breathing occurs naturally in the human body:

1) In the intermittent intervals between changeovers of the daily breathing.

2) At a heightened point of the transformational experience of the sexual act. (Breath is internalized in this act and therefore, the body is more focused and vitally charged than any other daily behaviour).

3) When a person is in deep sleep (the disappearance of the notion of the self in sleep is associated with middle path breathing).

4) As the last breath a person takes before death.

Human breathing will be centralised and mostly internalised when there are intense experiences in life like sexual intercourse, deep sleep and death. *Restoration of breath*, as a technique uses the middle path breathing to internalise breathing intentionally to achieve *Samadhi*, a state of pure consciousness. Middle path breathing as internalisation goes beyond experiencing the daily mode of time. Middle path breathing or *sushumna* in *yogic* terms, in this sense, destroys the individual consciousness of daily modes of time while extending it into timeless infinity. According to the *Sangitaratnakara*, the vital breath moving through the left and right nostrils indicates the movement of time, but the middle path breathing, the *susumna*, destroys time (153 c-155b).[67] The disappearance of the normal breathing through nostrils through internalisation and the disappearance of time (*kala*), according to the *Sangitaratnakara* arise from a particular use of breathing technique, which is the rise of internalised breath from the lower tip of the vertebral column up to the thousand-petalled cerebral aperture. As the text further says, "the 'duality' ceases and there is only oneness in consciousness... [in which] time transcends in eternity."[68] In my research, this technique can only be explained through the *Restoration of breath.*

Restoration of breath is an approach to breath. It denotes a particular system of breathing. It invokes an upward and downward movement of breath within the internal channels without any outward trace: the two other nostril modes, the left and the right are absent when you re-store breath. There is a constant flow of air within the internal system, but it is not perceptible to the sensory perceptions of an observer. In this sense, you cannot feel and measure the outer flow of the air when restoration of breath is in operation. *Restoration of breath* is the sole base of the *Siddha Yoga* practice of meditation, which is introduced by Swami Shivananda Paramhamsa.[69]

Restoration of breath is part of twenty-four patterns of sequential breathing known as *Gati,* which literally means directions. This system offers twenty-four patterns of breath directions consisting mostly of the sounds of birds and animals, which vibrate at different parts of the body. Out of these twenty-four patterns, eighteen are to do with a convenient sitting position and the remaining 6 are to do with bodily movements. Both are intended to create very high energy levels in the body. This breathing system is practised by people who belong to the *Siddha* lineage.[70] Restoration of breath is said to be the practice through which the state of *Samadhi* or pure consciousness is attained. Let me explain the system through the following drawings. Each line describes six distinct patterns of breathing. The directions of the breath's flow are marked by arrows. Here is the first line with the first set of patterns.

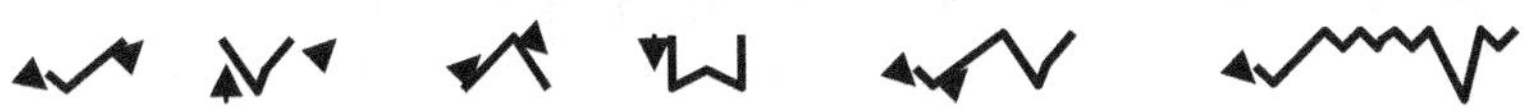

Siddha Yoga prescribes that the first set of six patterns of breathing is to be practised for one hour in the morning from 3am to 4am, with ten minutes for each pattern of breathing.

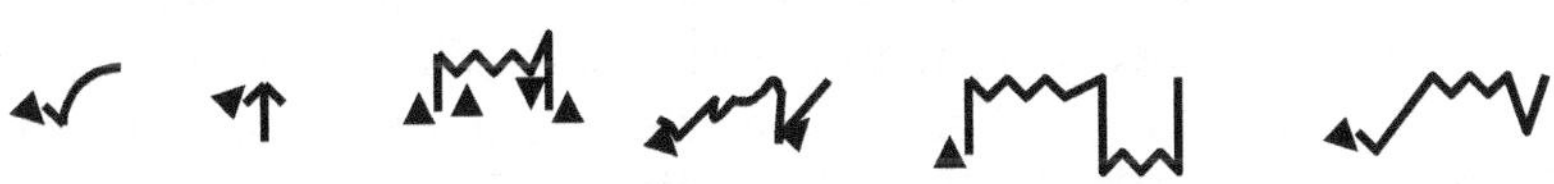

The second set of another six patterns is to be practiced between 12 noon to 1pm every day, also with 10 minutes for each pattern of breath.

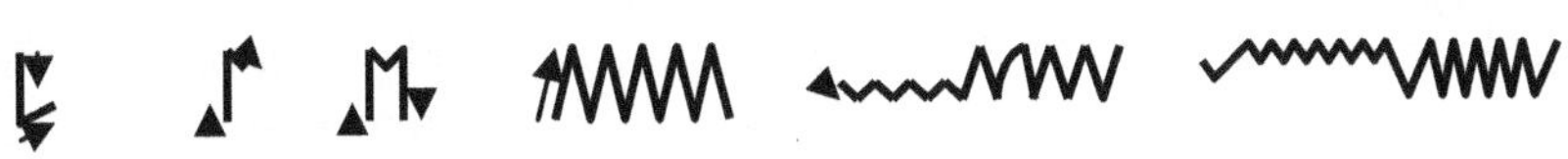

The third set also consists of 6 patterns of breathing, which is to be practised from 7.30pm to 8.30 pm every day. The eighteen patterns of breathing illustrated in the above three lines or sets are to be carried out only in a sitting position.

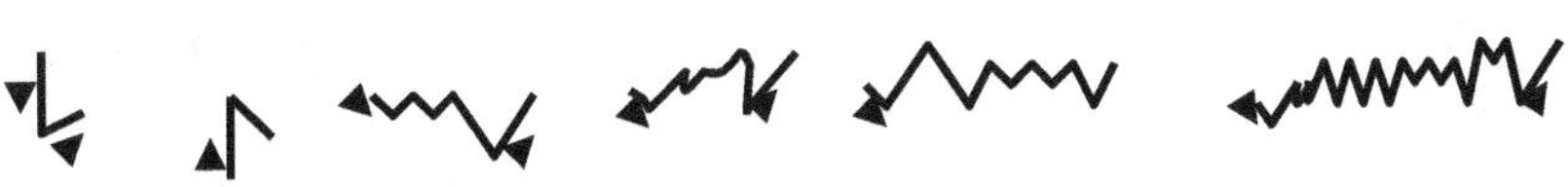

The fourth and the final set also includes six patterns of breathing, however, they can only be carried out along with movements. This is called *nadanam* or the dance, also known as the *dance of Shiva* in delight in which breathing co-exists with movements. According to Guru Rajendra Siddha Yogi, this is a state of absolute 'solitude' with the 'delight' of 'dancing' united in a single thread of awareness in which the bodily activities are profoundly focused and breath is properly internalised, which eventually alters level of consciousness.

Bharata's idea of Shiva as the first dancer and Brahma as the creator of the art of acting suggests the co-existence of meditation and performance as aspects of a single awareness which is the unity of consciousness. *Nadanam*, the dance, the fourth set, has to be practiced at the end of each set of patterns from one to three at 4am, 1pm and 8.30pm. *Siddha Yoga* strongly suggests that the internalisation of breathing through the *restoration of breath* is the fundamental technique to achieve highest form of human consciousness.

How does the practice of *restoration of breath* affect body, mind and consciousness? Body and mind are not two separate entities according to *Siddha Yoga*. Rather, these are considered as material elements presented in the body through respiration of breath. Breath is the physical counterpart of mind. All sensory and motor functions of the body are performed with the help of breath. Thus, breath is mind in action: the movement of breath is the movement of the body as well as that of the mind. The body is the basis of all experiences and the mind is something which is experienced in the body. Similarly, our knowledge of the world is experienced through the physical faculties of perception and the psychological functions of memory and re-cognition. Thus, breath links all psycho-physical functions of the body. *Restoration of breath* as a technique of internalising breath through the middle path is a way of understanding the existence of an altered level of individual awareness in which the aspects of knowing, knowledge and the knower are properly united.

Middle path breathing refers to a shift in time. The left and right path breathing suggest a conventional pattern of human respiration and a conventional sense of daily time. The middle path breathing, however, creates a shift in our daily perception and experience of time, through creating an infinite cosmic space and a different sense of time within. The daily modes of consciousness can be altered through middle path breathing by altering the mode of perceiving time. *Restoration of breath* is a movement upward and downward through the middle path which incorporates or unifies the other two modes, left and right, to create a timeless sense of infinitude and a field of vital energy within. This act of internalisation creates a shift in the individual perception of ordinary time by incorporating left and right nostril modes. In other words, the disappearance of left and right nostril modes brings a crucial shift in the individual's sense of time. *Restoration of breath* offers a technique to abandon the normal respiration using left and right nostrils. Breath is the physical counterpart of time incorporated in individual consciousness, and any shift taking place in the ordinary modes of breathing certainly will change the field of consciousness. *Restoration of breath* in this sense is a technical device invented to allow the practitioner to go beyond ordinary space-time parameters to change the state of consciousness, from daily to extra-daily, where extra-daily implies a higher state of consciousness, as discussed at the beginning of this chapter.

4.6 Performing Breath: *Santarasa*

Abhinavagupta introduced *santarasa*, firstly, as an extension of his philosophical enquiries in the field of theatre and secondly, as an explanation of his spiritual practice, which is based on the Tantric Saivism of Kashmir. Let us look at the concept and the consciousness background of *santarasa*. According to the Samkhya theory of *pancham-kosha*, the knowing self consists of five layers: *annamaya kosa* (the gross anatomical base), *pranamaya kosa* (the breath base), *manomaya kosa* (the emotive base), *vijnanamaya kosa* (the knowledge base) and finally, the *anandamaya kosa* (the delight base). All sensory perceptions, passive or active, filter through these various layers. Knowledge is the source of *ananda,* the joy or delight, according to the Indian theory of cognition; knowledge arising from experience has the potential of altering the conditions of knowing the Self from the narrow boundaries of the daily perceptual realities. *Anandamayakosa,* the delight base, is regarded as the highest state of individual consciousness and to enable an experience of this *ananda,* the delight, is the purpose of both art and spirituality. *Turiya* and *rasa*, in this sense, are regarded as the same experience of a higher state of consciousness experienced through the practices of meditation or art.

The transformation of consciousness towards altered states through perception and experience of the perceiver is the most focused area of debate in Indian aesthetics. Abhinavagupta describes this process by using a phrase *sattva-udreka*, which means the 'arising of *sattva*'- the arising of pure essence.[71] He explains it as a state of equanimity beyond perception, emotion and knowledge, and further explains it as an altered state of consciousness, which forms the basis of his *santa rasa*, a state of *pure experience* beyond contemplation. Being in this state is *ananda* and the ultimate goal of art, according to Indian aesthetic views, is to bring this experience to the 'beholders'. In Sankara, the great seventh century commentator of *Advaita Vedanta*, we see the philosophical implications of this concept presented in two of his compositions called *Saundaryalahari* (The Ecstasy of Beauty) and *Anandalahari* (The Ecstasy of Delight). *Anandalahari* consists of forty-one verses discussing the issues of intellect and spirit whereas *Saundaryalahari* describes aspects of female beauty in detail through fifty-nine verses. While describing the beauty of *Tripurasundari,* the female goddess of the Sakti cult, Sankara transfigures the extreme physical beauty into devotion, an equanimity of a different kind. Sankara evokes lust but the entire focus is to bring the divine, and this is the basic idea from which Abhinavagupta develops his theory on *santa rasa*.

Bharata mentions eight *rasas* in the *Natyasastra* as the erotic, comic, pathetic, furious, heroic, terrible, odious and marvellous. Abhinavagupta adds a ninth rasa.

> Santa, which has sama for its *sthayibhava,* leads to *moksha,* arises from *vibhavs* such as knowledge of the truth, detachment, purity of mind etc. It should be acted out by the *anubhava* such as *yama* and *niyama,* meditation on the Self, concentration of the mind on the self (*dharana*), devotion (*upasana*), compassion towards all creatures, and the wearing of religious paraphernalia (*lingagrahana*). …*Santarasa* has been taught as a means to the highest happiness. It arises from a desire to secure the liberation of the Self and leads to knowledge of the truth. ..*Santarasa* is that state wherein one feels the same towards all creatures, wherein there is no pain, no happiness, no hatred and no envy. *Santa* is one's natural state of mind (*prakrti*). Other emotions such as love etc. are deformations of that original state.[72]

This illustration of the nature of *santarasa* clearly establishes the links between *rasa*, aesthetic delight, and pure consciousness. The level of consciousness experienced in *santarasa* is equivalent to *Turiya* or pure consciousness. Perhaps one difference might be that the experience of *rasa* enabled for the spectator during a performance is lost when the spectator returns to ordinary life after the performance ends, whereas *Turiya* is permanent; repeated exposure to the experience of *rasa*, however, should help develop higher states of consciousness and, the eventually permanent experience of *Turiya*.

Sankara and Abhinavagupta emphasise a similar kind of a higher state of consciousness as the goal of spiritual practice as well as the practice of art. A parallel reading of Sankara and Abhinavagupta in the context of *Advaita* philosophy and art will certainly offer new insights into the issues of consciousness and *rasa*. According to Sankara, the *yogi* combines the mundane and divine into *samadhi*, a state of modified consciousness of non-dual existence. It is a state of freedom from the bondages of temporal limitations of here and now. As William M. Indich examines the *Advaita* model of consciousness, two approaches, theoretical and practical, exist in understanding the higher states of consciousness (Indich 2000, 65). The theoretical approach shows the interiorization and unification of consciousness and the practical approach suggests the methods to achieve that level of experience. *Advaita* offers the theoretical understanding and *Yoga* offers the practical methods. Sankara's and Abhinavagupta's philosophies and aesthetic views combined these elements and became one of the most developed traditions of thought in Indian philosophy. According to this view, performance became a form of meditation by exploring *santarasa* because *santa* as a *rasa* refers to a neutral state of consciousness placed within the 'gap' between inbreath and outbreath. In chapter 3, I described breath-related training available in *Kudiyattam* with each rasa. In addition to the material presented there, I checked the breathing of Usha Nangiyar when she performs *santarasa* and it was evident that breath disappears during her acting of *santarasa* as is the case with *restoration of breath* technique in *Siddha Yoga*.

Summary

Consciousness can be understood as patterns of spatio-temporal relations operating within the fields of human cognition through individual perception and experience. Consciousness, in this ordinary sense, is the awareness of the stream of events passing through individual perception, which is embedded in spatio-temporal parameters. The term *repetition* clearly establishes the fundamental links between time and consciousness in the acts of reading including literary and artistic representations. There are further levels of individual consciousness that are presented by Plotinus as a merging into timeless infinitude in which individual mind, ego, object worlds and subject-object cognition all drop away. *Advaita Vedanta* philosophy of India and various *yogic* traditions offer various models of this higher level of individual development. In most of these fully developed systems of thought, consciousness appears as the state of awareness beyond the level of ordinary time. This state is explained as the 'timeless infinitude' or a state in which 'silence co-exists with activity'. In Kashmir Saivism, breath, time and consciousness are interconnected in the sense that breath is the physical counterpart of time and by altering this flow of breath/time a 'gap' in the stream of consciousness can be created, which is, largely, explained as the timeless infinitude and the 'outside' of perception and meaning. *Siddha Yoga* of South India, particularly, offers a practice called *Restoration of Breath* through which this 'gap' can be identified as an extension or alteration of daily consciousness. This 'gap' is located in between inbreath and outbreath, and outbreath and inbreath. *Restoration of breath* is a technique to identify and explore this 'gap' located in the physical flow of breath/time. Finally, *Santarasa* produces a similar level of consciousness in performance and practices of this can be found in *Kudiyattam*.

The chapter, therefore, suggests that performance and meditation are two psychophysical techniques that alter individual consciousness in different ways in order to experience the same level of consciousness which exists beyond the ordinary spatio-temporal dimensions of waking and dreaming states of consciousness. The chapter, thus, concludes that breath being the physical counterpart of *time* present in the body is an effective tool, initially, to explore actors dormant energy level of the body and secondly, to alter the field of the awareness of consciousness from daily to extra-daily. Cessation of breath, on the contrary, creates pause in this flow of the endless identification of signifiers. When breath stops time stops. When time stops there is a 'gap' in the chain of the presence of signifiers that we experience as daily. This 'gap' is a different perceptual modality, which is neutral in Zero velocity. It accelerates without succession and vibrates without movement. It is an alteration of consciousness, and any alteration of consciousness, intentional or unintentional, causes alteration in normal breathing. Breathing modes and patterns change according to the emotional and physical activities that we carry out in our daily life. This means that any intentional alteration of breathing, on the other hand, can alter individual consciousness: *Restoration of Breath* is a practical approach to this psychophysical experience of consciousness in which time exists only in eternity and void beyond memory and meaning.

Notes

[1]<http://en.wikibooks.org/wiki/Consciousness_studies:_The_description_of_consciousness> (consulted September 5, 2007)
[2] Ibid., p. 1.
[3] Peter Malekin and Ralph Yarrow, *Consciousness, Literature and Theatre: Theory and Beyond,* (London: Macmillan, 1997) p. 34.
[4] Peter Malekin, " Performance and Consciousness as Freedom" in *Performing Arts International,* vol.1, part, 4. p. 93-94.
[5]<http://en.wikibooks.org/wiki/Consciousness_studies:_The_description_of_consciousness> (consulted September 5, 2007)
[6] Ibid.
[7] Ibid.
[8] Ibid.
[9] Ralph Yarrow, *Indian Theatre: Theatre of Origin, Theatre of Freedom,* (London: Curzon, 2001), p. 5
[10]<http://en.wikipedia.org/wiki/jane_Roberts> (consulted September 5, 2007).
[11] Peter Malekin and Ralph Yarrow, *Consciousness, Literature and Theatre: Theory and Beyond,* (London: Macmillan, 1997) p. 37.
[12] Ibid., p. 38.
[13] Ibid., p. 38.
[14] Ibid., p. 38.
[15] Peter Malekin, "Performance and Consciousness as Freedom" in *Performing Arts International,* vol.1, part, 4. p. 97.
[16] Ibid., p. 97.
[17] K.P. Narayana Pisharoti, (tr.), *Bharatamuniyude Natyasastram*, vol.1, (Trichur: Kerala Sahitya Akademi, 1987) p. 79. This edition of the book is only available in Malayalam, the regional language of Kerala and I use this for my references for the entire thesis. The author has translated the book directly from the various available Sanskrit manuscripts to the regional language. Since the author can not read or write English, he was not influenced by other editions translated in English. So, this edition is an authentic version of *The Natyasastra* available in Sanskrit.
[18] Peter Malekin, "Performance and Consciousness as Freedom" in *Performing Arts International,* vol.1, part, 4. p. 98. What Malekin explains here is the concepts of *Nada* and *Bindu* presented elaborately in various classical Indian texts of spirituality and mysticism. *Nada*, the sound emerges from *Bindu*, the static infinitude, and space and time are born out of this subtle exploration. See ch.2 for further details.
[19] Ralph Yarrow, "Neutral Consciousness in the experience of Theatre" in Mosaic (Summer 1986) p. 2.
[20] Ibid., p. 3.
[21] Ibid., p. 8.
[22] Ibid., p. 8.
[23] Ibid., p. 9.
[24] Ibid., p. 9.
[25] Ibid., p. 10.
[26] Ibid., p. 11.

[27] Ibid., p. 11.
[28] Daniel Meyer-Dinkgräfe, *Consciousness and The Actor*, (Frankfurt: Peter Lang, 1996) p. 125-134.
[29] Ibid., p. 127.
[30] Alexander: 1986, p. 295, in Meyer-Dinkgräfe, 1996, p. 30
[31] Alexander, 1989, p. 355, in Ibid., p. 30.
[32] Ibid., p. 133.
[33] Ibid., p. 133.
[34] Quoted in Meyer-Dinkgräfe, Ibid., 1996, p. 133.
[35] Ibid., p. 126.
[36] Arne Melberg, *Theories of Memesis,* (Cambridge: Cambridge University Press, 1995), p. 141.
[37] Ibid., p. 23.
[38] Gerald F. Else, *Plato and Aristotle on Poetry,* (Chapel Hill: NC, 1986), p. 74.
[39] Arne Melberg, *Theories of Mimesis,* (Cambridge: Cambridge University Press, 1995), p. 44-45.
[40] Paul Ricoeur, *Time and Narrative,* tr. K. McLaughlin & D. Pellaure, (Chicago University Press, 1984), vol. 1, p. 31.
[41] Ibid, p. 3.
[42] Kierkegaard, *Repetition: An Essay in Experimental Psychology,* tr. Walter Lowrie, (New York: Evanston & London: Harper & Row, 1964), p. 33.
[43] Michael Foucault, "Theatrum Philosophicum" in Timothy Murray, (ed.) *Mimesis, Masochism and Mime: The Politics of Theatricality in Contemporary French Thought,* (Michigan University Press, 1997), p. 216-238.
[44] Gilles Deleuze, *Difference and Repetition,* (London: Continuum, 2001), p. 8-16.
[45] Ibid., p. 16.
[46] Luce Irigaray, *The forgetting of Air in Martin Heidegger,* (London: Athlone, 1999), p. 164.
[47] Martin Heidegger, *An Introduction to Metaphysics,*(tr.) Ralph Manheim, (New Delhi: Motilal Banarsidass, 1999), p,4.
[48] Luce Irigaray, *The forgetting of Air in Martin Heidegger,* (London: Athlone, 1999), p. 8-9
[49] Ibid., p. 11.
[50] Antonin Artaud, *The Theatre and Its Double*, (London: Calder, 1989), p. 93.
[51] Ibid., p. 89.
[52] Ibid., p. 93.
[53] Ibid., p. 92.
[54] See Chapter two for further details.
[55] Ibid., p. 92.
[56] Maharishi Mahesh Yogi, c.f. Daniel Meyer-Dinkgräfe, *Consciousness and the Actor,* (Frankfurt: Peter Lang, 1996), p. 153
[57] Antonin Artaud, *The Theatre and Its Double*, (London: Calder, 1989), p. 95.
[58] See Chapter three for more details.
[59] Bettina Bäumer, "Sun, Consciousness and Time: The way of Time and the Timeless in Kashmir Saivism" in Kapila Vatsyayan, ed. *Concept of Time Ancient and Modern,* (New Delhi: Indira Gandhi National Centre for the Arts, 1996) p. 73-77.
[60] Tantraloka: VII. 62-63

[61] Ibid., p. 73.
[62] TAI, VI. 179-180.
[63] L. Silburn, *Hymnes aux Kali,* Paris, 1975, p. 50.
[64] Bettina Bäumer, p. 75
[65] Tantraloka: VII.21-25
[66] See Chapter two for more details
[67] K.R. Shringy and Prem Lata Sharma, (tr.), *Sangitaratnakara of Sarngadevs,* vol.1, (New Delhi: Munshiram Manoharlal, 1991), p. 102.
[68] Ibid., p. 102.
[69] See Chapter 2.5.3 for the detailed description of the practice
[70] See Chapter two section 2.5 for more details.
[71] Haresh V. Dehejia, Makarand Paranjape, (ed.) *Saundarya: The Perception and Practice of Beauty in India.* New Delhi: Samvad India Foundation, 2003. p. 9.
[72] quoted in Meyer-Dinkgräfe, 1996. p. 145.

Conclusion

The point of departure for my argument in this book was the desire to explore the role of breath in relation to acting and actor training. I identified the need for this discussion from the insight that while many philosophers and theatre artists note the importance of the human body for life in general and in the contexts of performativity, theatricality, performance and theatre in particular, only very few note the relevance of one particular aspect of the body: breath. Related to that insight is my unique access, through my family, to specific aspects of Indian traditional knowledge that are explicitly related to breath. In Chapter one I demonstrated how the related concepts of performativity and theatricality are bound to notions of embodiment, but predominantly without reference to breath. The writings of Irigaray and Artaud are the exceptions. Chapter one concluded that breath in relation to theatre needs further attention. In Chapter two I described in detail how selected and relevant schools of thought in the West and in the East understand, describe and define breath. In Chapter three I analysed to what extent, if at all, different Western and Eastern approaches to actor training integrate breath-related techniques and how breath has been excluded in the major system of actor training in contemporary theatre. In Chapter four, I finally related techniques of breath to states and levels of consciousness and discussed how breath related techniques in the context of theatre can serve to develop altered states of consciousness. Below I will now summarise my findings.

Restoration of Breath, as an ancient technique found in the South Indian *Siddha* tradition, offers a clear and concrete understanding of breath as the key material element in the body. As such, breath is a transformative tool to extra-daily alterations in human consciousness. I have discussed the importance of breath in relevant performance, medical and spiritual schools and systems of traditional knowledge in India: the *Upanishads*, *Yoga*, *Tantra*, *Ayurveda* and *Marma* medicine. As a result of this discussion, breath is now understood as a psycho-physical tool, which is capable to alter the individual consciousness from daily to extra-daily. In the *Tantraloka,* for example, Abhinavagupta establishes the link between breath and consciousness by introducing the concept of *Kāla, time*. Traditional Indian philosophical thinking thus establishes the role of breath: breath represents the link between time and consciousness. Nostril modes change according to the type of the mental state and emotional texture. Similarly, the quality of individual awareness can also be changed by employing specific breathing techniques. According to South Indian *Siddha* tradition, these alterations of breathing are a vital source of energy transformations in the body firstly because breath is the vital substance of the body and therefore, vital physical energy can be manipulated by exploring breath. Secondly, nostril modes are connected to the individual's consciousness in the context of *time*; therefore, *Siddha Yoga* suggests systematic approaches to changing nostril modes in order to access an extra-daily sense of consciousness which is also named as *samadhi* or *turiya,* pure consciousness: this level of consciousness is beyond the daily sense of time. In this lies the significance of *restoration of breath* as a psycho-physical technique. The complete internalization of breathing called *restoration of breath* is further to the twenty-four patterns explained in Chapter Four, and a careful application of this technique creates a state of absolute coordination between mind and body by stepping out of the daily sense of time. *Restoration of Breath*, in this sense, offers a closure, an epistemological understanding and a practical approach, to the issues of mind-body duality in the contemporary debate.

Abhinavagupta established the links between breath and pure consciousness in *Tantraloka* as the highest state of spiritual achievement. He refers to a term *kālādhvan*, which is a technique through which pure consciousness can be experienced. Abhinavagupta's descriptions of the technique in *Tantraloka* do not seem to be offering any clear idea about the practice. However, my research shows that *kālādhvan* and *restoration of breath* are referring to a similar practice of internalising breath. Another reason for this conclusion is historical, in the sense that both the techniques, *kālādhvan* and *restoration of breath*, come from the Siva spiritual tradition. Abhinavagupta also introduced *santarasa* as the final state of acting *rasa* in a performance situation. As we see in Chapter four, Abhinavagupta explained *santarasa* as the rising of pure consciousness. On the basis of Sankara's *Advaita Vedanta* philosophy, Abhinavagupta explains *Santarasa* as a state of equanimity beyond perception, emotion and knowledge. *Santarasa,* in this sense, is an altered state of *pure experience* beyond contemplation. I cannot find any evidence that Abhinavagupta establishes a link between *santarasa* and breath as he does with pure consciousness and breath. However, *Kudiyattam* offers examples of the links between breath and *santarasa.* I have provided a detailed description of how *Kudiyattam* incorporates breathing techniques in training and performance in Chapter three: rasa acting in *Kudiyattam* shows the systematic applications of breath in acting. Breath is also applied to eye training in *Kudiyattam.* In this context, I have also demonstrated the origins of *Svara-vayu*, a highly important technique which incorporates breath in acting in *Kudiyattam* which has been lost in the course of time in Indian music and *Siddha Veda* traditions.

In this book I have not discussed the potential significance of *restoration of breath* and the breath-related training methods of *Kudiyattam* for future actor training. This is mainly because that research requires practice-based laboratory work investigating traditional material, *restoration of breath* and *Kudiyattam*, and their effects in training the body-mind of a contemporary actor. This book is only the beginning of a long-term research project that will establish a new phase in contemporary actor training—consciousness-related actor training.

Bibliography

Aristotle. 1936. *Aristotle on the Soul: Prava Naturalia, On breath.* (tr. Hett.W.S.) London: William Heinemann Ltd & Harvard University Press.

Artaud, Antonin. 1970. *Theatre andIts Double.* (tr. Corti, Victor) London: Calder & Boyars.

Awasthi, Suresh. 2001. *Performance Tradition in India.* New Delhi: National Book Trust.

Bäumer, Bettina. 1996. "Sun, Consciousness and Time: The way of Time and the Timeless in Kashmir Saivism" in *Concept of Time Ancient and Modern,* ed. Vatsyayan, Kapila. New Delhi: Indira Gandhi National Centre for the Arts: 73-77.

Berry, Cicely. 2000. *Voice and the Actor.* London: Virgin Books.

Brahmachari, Dhirendra. 1956. *Yogic Suksma Vyayama.* New Delhi: Dhirendra Yoga Publications.

Bhaskaran Nair, Thiruvallam. 1976. *Thirumandiram Moovariram.* Trivandrum: Kerala Vidya Peth.

Capra, Fritjof. 1981. *The Tao of Physics.* London: Fontana/Collins.

Chakravarti, Pulinbihari. 1975. *Origin and Development of the Samkhya System of Thought.* London: Luzac & Co, Ltd.

Dasgupta, Surendranath. 1955. *A History of Indian Philosophy.* Vol. 5. Cambridge: Cambridge University Press.

Davis, C. Tracy and Postlewait, Thomas (eds). 2003. *Theatricality.* Cambridge: Cambridge University Press.

Dehejia, V. Haresh and Paranjape, Makarand (ed.). 2003. *Saundarya: The Perception and Practice of Beauty in India.* New Delhi: Samvad India Foundation.

Deleuze, Gilles. 1990. *The Logic of Sense.* (tr. Mark Lester, with Charles Stivale) Constantin V. Boundas.(ed). New York: Columbia University Press.

——. 2001. *Difference and Repetition.* London & New York: Continuum.

De Man, Paul. 1979. *Allegories of Reading: Figural Language in Rousseau,Nietzsche, Rilke and Proust.* New Haven, Conn; London: Yale University Press.

Derrida, Jacques. 1982. *Margins of Philosophy.* (tr. Bass, Alan). Chicago: The University of Chicago Press.

——. 1997. "The Theatre of Cruelty and the Closure of Representation" in Timothy Murray (ed.) *Mimesis, Masochism and Mime: The Politics of Theatricality in Contemporary French Thought.* Ann Arbor: Michigan University Press: 40-62.

Eliade, Mircea. 1969. *Yoga: Immortality and Freedom.* (tr. R. Trask, Willard) Princeton: Princeton University Press.

Else, F. Gerald. 1986. (ed). *Plato and Aristotle on Poetry.* Chapel Hill; London: University of North Carolina Press.

Fischer-Lichte, Erika. 1997. "Theatricality", in *Theatre Research International.* 20 (2): 218-260.

Foucault, Michel. 1997. "*Theatrum Philosophicum",* in Timothy Murray (ed) *Mimesis, Masochism and Mime: The Politics of Theatricality in Contemporary French Thought.* Ann Arbor: Michigan University Press: 216-238.

Grant, Sara. 1999. *Sankaracarya's Concept of Relation.* New Delhi: Motilal Banarsidass.

Grotowski, Jerzy. 1991. *Towards a Poor Theatre.* London: Methuen.

Halbfass, Wilhelm. "*Space or Matter: The Concept of Akāsa in Indian Thought*", Rabindranath Tagore Lecture, Centre for Philosophy and Foundations of Science, New Delhi: 1999.

Heidegger, Martin. 1999. *An Introduction to Metaphysics.* (tr. Ralph Manheim) New Delhi: Motilal Banarsidass.

——. 1993. "The End of Philosophy and the Task of Thinking" in David Farrell Krell (tr.) *Basic Writings.* New York: Harper Collins: 427-449

H. Ittelson, William. 1960. *Visual Space Perception.* New York: Springer Publishing Company.

Hodge, Alison. (ed). 2000. *Twentieth Century Actor Training.* London & New York: Routledge.

Irigaray, Luce. 1999. *The Forgetting of Air in Martin Heidegger.* (tr. Mary Beth Mader). London: Athlone Press.

——. 2002. *Between East and West.* New York: Columbia University Press.

Iyengar, B.S.K. 2000. *Light on Yoga.* New Delhi: Harper Collins.

James Larson, Gerald and Shankar Bhattacharya, Ram. 1987. (eds). *Sāmkhya:A Dualist Tradition in Indian Philosophy.* Princeton: Princeton University Press.

Johari, Harish. 1989. *Breath, Mind and Consciousness.* Rochester & Vermont: Destiny Books.

Karunakaran Vaidyar, Kaimanam. 2002. *Marmasastra Patangal.* Trivandrum: Published by the author.

Kierkegaard, Søren. 1964. *Repetition: An Essay in Experimental Psychology.* (tr. Walter Lowrie) New York: Evanston & London: Harper & Row.

Kochukrishnan Nadar. K. Kanjiramkulam. 1968. *Marmasastra Samāhāram.* Trivandrum: Deshabhivardhini Publishing House.

Lecoq, Jacques. 2000. *The Moving Body: Teaching Creative Theatre.* London: Methuen.

Madhava Chakyar, Ammannur. 1995. "My Training, My Gurus" in *Sangeet Natak,* (Special issue), no. 111-114: 141-146.

Madhava Chakyar, Mani. 1995. "The Training Methods of Kudiyattam", in *Sangeet Natak,* (special issue), no. 111-114: 48- 54.

Malekin, Peter. 1999. "Performance and Consciousness as Freedom", In *Performing Arts International,* vol. 1(4): 93-101.

Malekin, Peter & Yarrow, Ralph. 1997. *Consciousness, Literature and Theatre: Theory and Beyond.* London: Macmillan Press.

Martin, John. 2004. *The Intercultural Performance Handbook.* London: Routledge.

Melberg, Arne. 1995. *Theories of Mimesis.* Cambridge: Cambridge University Press.

Meyer Dinkgräfe, Daniel. 1996. *Consciousness and the Actor.* Frankfurt: Peter Lang.

——. 1999. "Consciousness and the Concept of Rasa", *Performing Arts Journal,* 1(4): 103-115.

——. 2001. *Approaches to Acting: Past and Present.* London & New York: Continuum.

Nair, D. Appukuttan. 1995. "Kudiyattam and Bhasa" in *Sangeet Natak,* (Special issue), no. 111-114: 190-194.

Nair, T. K. Ramunni. 1955. *Natyarcana.* Calicut: P.K. Brothers.

Narayana Pisharoti, K.P. 1987. (tr.). *Bharatamuniyude Natyasastram*. vol.1, Trichur: Kerala Sahitya Akademi.

Núñez, Nicolas. 1996. *Anthropocosmic Theatre*. Amsterdam: Harwood.

Oida, Yoshi. 1997. *The Invisible Actor*. London: Methuen.

Patton, Paul. 2000. *Deleuze and the Political*. London: Routledge.

Phelan, Peggy. 1993. *Unmarked: the Politics of Performance*. London & New York: Routledge.

Prabhavananda, Swami and Manchester, Frederick. 1971. *The Upanishads: Breath of the Eternal*. California: Vedanta Press.

Ramacharaka, Yogi. 1960. *Science of Breath*. London: Fowler.

Renfrew Brooks, Douglas (ed). 2000. *Meditation Revolution: A History and Theology of the Siddha Yoga Lineage*. New Delhi: Motilal Banarsidass.

Ricoeur, Paul. 1984. *Time and Narrative*. (tr. McLaughlin, K & Pellaure, D.) Chicago University Press, vol. 1.

Roach, Joseph R. 1999. *The Player's Passion: Studies in the Science of Acting*. Ann Arbor: University of Michigan Press.

Sauter, Willmar. 2000. *The Theatrical Event: Dynamics of Performance and Perception*. Iowa City: University of Iowa Press.

——. 1991. "Who Is Who and What Is What? Introductory Notes," in *Advances in Reception and Audience Research,* 2: 5-16.

Schechner, Richard. 2002. *Performance Studies: An Introduction*. London & New York: Routledge.

Schumacher, Claude with Singleton, Brian. 2001. (ed.). *Artaud on Theatre*. London: Methuen.

Shivananda Paramahamsar, Swami. 1922. *Siddha Veda*. Kerala: Siddha Samajam.

Shringy, R. K. and Sharma, Prem Lata. 1991. *Sangitaratnakara of Sarngadeva*. (tr.) vol. 1, New Delhi: Munshiram Manoharlal.

Sivapriyananda, Swami. 1996. *Secret Power of Tantrik Breathing*. New Delhi: Abhinav Publications.

Vatsyayan, Kapila (ed.). 1996. *Concept of Time Ancient and Modern,* New Delhi: Indira Gandhi National Centre for the Arts.

Venu, G. 1995. "Swaravayu: A Unique Method of Breath-Control", in *Sruti: Music & Dance Magazine,* 125: 45.

Yarrow, Ralph. 2001. *Indian Theatre: Theatre of Origin, Theatre of Freedom*. London: Curzon.

——. 1986. "Neutral Consciousness in the experience of Theatre". *Mosaic*, 19(3): 1-13.

Wildish, Paul. 2000. *The Book of Ch'i*. Boston: Journey Editions.

Woodroffe, Sir John. 2001. *The Garland of Letters*. Madras: Ganesh & Co.

Zarrilli, Phillip. 1995. "On the Edge of A Breath, Looking", in Phillip Zarrilli (ed.) *Acting (Re)Considered*. London: Routledge.

Websites:

http://kh.bu.edu/artwithbraininmind-1/1736.html (consulted July 12, 2007)

http://plato.stanford.edu/entries/descartes-epistemology/4 (consulted March 12, 2005)

http://en.wikibooks.org/wiki/Consciousness_studies:_The_description_of_consciousness (consulted September 5, 2007)

http://en.wikipedia.org/wiki/jane_Roberts (consulted September 5, 2007)